Mounir HAGUI

The emergency medical service (SAMU)

AF301087

Mounir HAGUI

The emergency medical service (SAMU)

Diagnostic performance analysis

ScienciaScripts

Imprint

Any brand names and product names mentioned in this book are subject to trademark, brand or patent protection and are trademarks or registered trademarks of their respective holders. The use of brand names, product names, common names, trade names, product descriptions etc. even without a particular marking in this work is in no way to be construed to mean that such names may be regarded as unrestricted in respect of trademark and brand protection legislation and could thus be used by anyone.

Cover image: www.ingimage.com

This book is a translation from the original published under ISBN 978-620-6-72412-4.

Publisher:
Sciencia Scripts
is a trademark of
Dodo Books Indian Ocean Ltd. and OmniScriptum S.R.L publishing group

120 High Road, East Finchley, London, N2 9ED, United Kingdom
Str. Armeneasca 28/1, office 1, Chisinau MD-2012, Republic of Moldova, Europe
Printed at: see last page
ISBN: 978-620-8-33505-2

Copyright © Mounir HAGUI
Copyright © 2024 Dodo Books Indian Ocean Ltd. and OmniScriptum S.R.L publishing group

Contents

1 INTRODUCTON

The purpose of the emergency medical services (SAMU) is to organise help and provide the sick, injured and pregnant women, wherever they may be, with emergency care appropriate to their condition. Their mission is to provide a response to unplanned emergencies of varying degrees of seriousness, using resources that are limited compared with the diagnostic and therapeutic arsenal available in hospital.

The attending physician plays a crucial role when faced with an emergency call from a patient whose life could be at risk if appropriate care is not taken quickly and in the most appropriate way.

His role is to ensure that, by listening carefully to the patient's medical needs and asking precise questions from a distance, he is able to suspect a clinical diagnosis and initiate the response best suited to the nature of the situation.

The emergency doctor, who plays just as important a role as the regulating doctor, will go out via an emergency medical and resuscitation unit (SMUR) to treat a patient outside the hospital, based solely on the regulating doctor's diagnostic assumptions. At the scene, he or she will still have the task, with limited resources, of confirming or rectifying the preliminary clinical diagnosis, initiating medical treatment and deciding whether or not to evacuate the patient to an emergency facility for further treatment in consultation with the attending physician.

The conditions in which patients are treated in emergency departments are far superior, giving emergency doctors a certain degree of ease in their diagnostic and therapeutic approach. The diagnosis suggested by the attending doctor and suspected by the doctor on the scene is generally confirmed in the emergency department.

Our study is original in that we are interested in pre-hospital medicine, one of the strongest links in acute medicine. Few studies have focused on evaluating the diagnostic relevance of EMS/EMUR services in Tunisia.

The aim of our work is to assess the degree of concordance between the diagnosis suggested by the regulating doctor, the diagnosis suspected by the intervention doctor and the final diagnosis established by the emergency doctor used as a reference.

2 METHODS

1. Type and location of study

This is a prospective, observational, single-centre study conducted at the military emergency medical assistance centre (CMAMU) and the emergency reception service (SAU) of the main military training hospital in Tunis (HMPIT).

1.1. The Military Emergency Medical Assistance Centre (CMAMU)

The Military Emergency Medical Aid Centre (CMAMU) was created by ministerial decree No. 66/2013, dated 03 February 2013, which also governs its organisation and scope of action. The centre was inaugurated by the Tunisian Defence Minister on 14 June 2013 and has been operational ever since.

The CMAMU is located at the Tunis Military Training Hospital (HMPIT). Its premises include :

- The call reception and regulation unit (CRRA) with a toll-free number: 199
- Currently, it has only one mobile emergency and resuscitation service, the SMUR in Tunis, located at the HMPIT, the main military training hospital in Tunis, and comprising 2 mobile hospital units (UMH).
- A CESU emergency training and simulation centre
- Three administrative offices, 2 on-call rooms and an equipment shop.

The beneficiaries of care are military personnel, civilian civil servants and pensioners from the Ministry of Defence, as well as their families.

1.2. Role of the CMAMU

The CMAMU provides :

- Medical regulation throughout Tunisia. Constant medical monitoring means that the most appropriate medical response can be given as quickly as possible, and patients can be referred to the most appropriate hospital if necessary.
- A response function enabling victims to be rescued and resuscitated at the scene of the incident and transported to hospital.
- Initial and continuing medical training in the different areas of health and in the different specialities.
- Medical support for military and national events if required by ministerial order.

1.3. CMAMU staff

The CMAMU is under the direction of an associate professor of emergency medicine. The medical team is made up of 7 permanent doctors who provide :

- The functions of medical regulation and pre-hospital intervention on a 24-hour call-out basis.
- Ongoing training for the department's medical and paramedical staff.
- The development of working procedures and scientific work.

The paramedical team consists of :

- a supervisor
- 12 nurses who alternate between working as medical regulation assistants (ARM) and intervention nurses.
- 1 medical secretary
- 1 surface technician

The CMAMU receives an average of 400,000 calls a year, including 1,171 regulatory cases and 619 emergency medical services (data for 2018).

2. Duration of the study

The study was carried out over a 12-month period in 2018.

3. Study objectives

The main objective of our study was to assess the degree of overall diagnostic agreement between the regulating physician, the interventional physician and the emergency physician. The secondary objective was to compare, by disease group, the different diagnoses suggested by the regulating doctor, suspected by the intervention doctor and confirmed by the emergency doctor.

4. Patients

4.1. Inclusion criteria

The study included all adult patients over 18 years of age for whom an EMS discharge had been decided by the attending physician, who had been attended by an emergency physician at the scene and subsequently transferred to the HMPIT emergency department.

4.2. Non-inclusion criteria

Patients with the following characteristics were not included in the study:

- Pregnant women with a reason for calling in relation to their pregnancy.
- Any traumatic pathology resulting from an accident or assault
- Secondary transfers
- Deaths and cardio-respiratory arrests at the scene
- Deliberate or accidental drug intoxication, the diagnosis of which is confirmed by anamnesis of the regulations.
- Non-medical discharge by a nurse or emergency medical technician.

4.3. Exclusion criteria

Patients who were rapidly redirected to an inpatient department even before starting emergency care, and cases with missing data that could affect the relevance of the study, were excluded from the study.

4.4. Judging criteria

In our study, we limited ourselves to two qualitative evaluation parameters:

- **Primary endpoint:** The diagnostic performance of the military emergency medical aid centre, comparing the diagnosis made in the pre-hospital setting by the regulating and intervention doctors with that made by the reference emergency doctor.
- **Secondary endpoint:** Decision-making performance, by assessing the degree to which patients were prioritised according to clinical severity.

5. Methods

5.1. Data collection

Data on the patients included in the study were extracted from the CMAMU centre's regulation and intervention forms and from patients' medical records in the emergency department of the main military hospital in Tunis.

Epidemiological, clinical and para-clinical, diagnostic and therapeutic data were collected using a Case Report Form (CRF) created and dedicated to the study (Appendix 1).

The CRF had 3 sections:

- *Section 1*: dedicated to the medical regulator, comprising :
- epidemiological data on patients
- evoked clinical and diagnostic data
- the degree of prioritisation according to the clinical classification of patients in the emergency medical services (R1, R2, R3 and R4) (Appendix 2,4)
- the degree of relevance of the diagnosis made by the regulatory physician.

- *Section 2*: dedicated to the intervention doctor including:
- suspected clinical and diagnostic findings

- on-site therapies
- the degree of urgency judged by the emergency doctor according to the clinical classification of illnesses in the CCMS emergency and resuscitation medical service (Appendix 5).

■ *Section 3*: dedicated to the emergency doctor including :
- the final diagnosis
- the final outcome for patients

5.2. Qualifications of regulating and intervention doctors

These are general practitioners working full-time at the military SAMU/SMUR centre with more than 5 years' experience.

6. Conduct of the study

The study was carried out throughout 2018, 24 hours a day. All patients eligible for the study were included by the regulating doctor, who completed part 1 of the CRF, and then transferred to the intervention doctor, who completed part 2 of the study. At the emergency department, the patient is admitted with his CRF, and the emergency doctor fills in section 3.

7. Data analysis

The data were analysed using SPSS version 19.0 software.

We have calculated :
- simple frequencies and relative frequencies, as well as percentages for qualitative variables.
- of means, medians and standard deviations for quantitative variables.
- The concordance study was carried out using Cohen's Kappa concordance test.

In all the statistical tests used, the significance level was set at 0.05.

8. Bibliographic research

French and English were used as research languages.

8.1. Databases used

Bibliographical research was carried out through :
- Search engines: Pubmed, Google scholar.
- The websites: Science direct, Hinari, Masson, Cochrane

Relevant articles, literature reviews and case studies have been referenced in this work.

The bibliography section of the websites of Tunisia's faculties of medicine was consulted to search for theses and dissertations.

8.2. Key words

The keywords used for the bibliographic search were :

Service d'aide medicale urgente : Service d'aide médicale urgente

Diagnosis : Diagnosis

Emergencies

Evaluation : Evaluation

Performance: Performance

8.3. Treatment of quotations and references

Version 5.0 of Zotero has been used to organise the references.

9. Declaration of no conflict of interest

We declare no conflict of interest between the author of this research, the supervisor and the various departments involved in the study. No subsidy was obtained for this work.

10. Ethical considerations, confidentiality and protection of patients' personal data

When this work was carried out, personal data enabling the identification of the individual was not revealed, and anonymity on the files and data collection forms was respected.

3 RESULTS

1. Patient recruitment

The study took place over a one-year period during 2018. The number of patients eligible for our study was 209.

Figure 1 illustrates the recruitment process for patients eligible for the study.

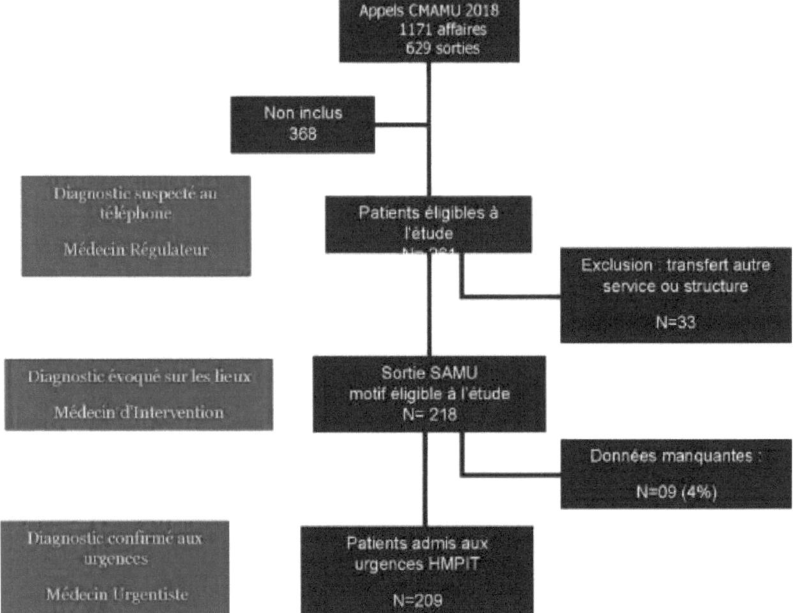

Figure 1: <u>Conduct of the study and patient inclusion</u>

2. Patient epidemiological data

2.1. Type

The patients were divided into 144 men (69%) and 65 women (31%), with a sex ratio of 2.21 (Figure 2).

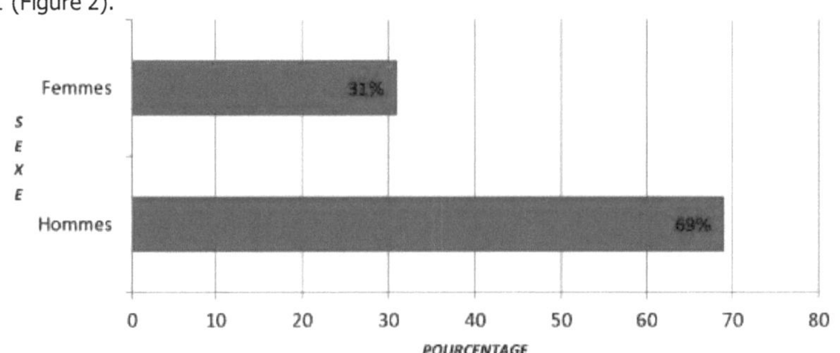

Figure 2: <u>Breakdown of patients by gender</u>

2.2. Age

The mean age was 51.2±35.6 years [16-88]. Half of the population studied (51%) was in the [40-60] age group. A third of patients (31%) were elderly (>60 years).

The breakdown by age group is shown in Figure 3.

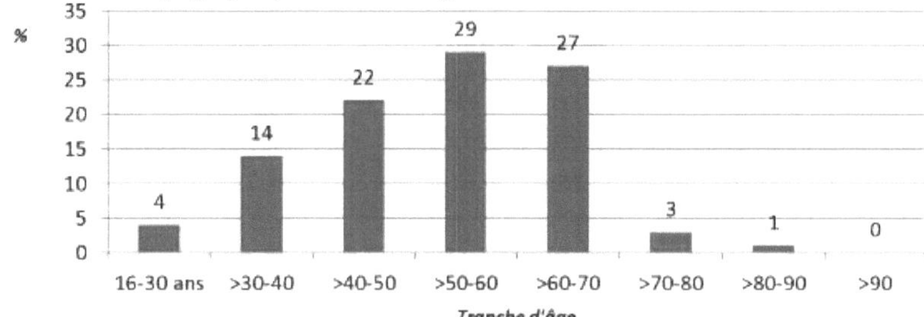

Figure 3: <u>Breakdown of patients by age in %.</u>

2.3. Administrative status and social security cover

In 65% of cases, the patient was a military pensioner or a member of a military family. The distribution of patients according to their administrative status is detailed in Table I :

<u>**Table I: Breakdown of patients by social security affiliation**</u>

Administrative status and social security cover	N	%
1. Military retirement	89	42,5
2. Military or civilian active in the armed forces	64	30,5
3. Military family	43	21
4. Civilian (CNSS and other)	12	6
Total	209	100%

2.4. Domiciliation of patients by governorate

The CMAMU's SMUR activity covered 1/3 of the Tunisian territory (8 governorates). Most of the SMUR discharges were made in the Greater Tunis region, with a rate of 86.5%. The breakdown of discharges by governorate is shown in Table II and Figure 4.

<u>**Table II: Breakdown of patients by place of residence**</u>

Governorate of origin	N =	%	
Greater Tunis	181	86,5	
Tunis	98	47	
Manouba	37	17,5	
Ariana	25	12	
Ben Arous	22	10	
Other Governorates	28	13,5	
Bizerte	16		7,5
Nabeul	9		4,5
Zaghouan	2		1
Jendouba	1	0,5	
Total	168		100%

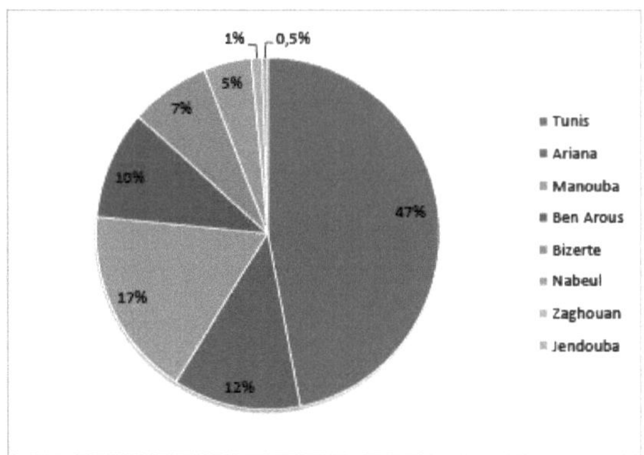

Figure 4: <u>Breakdown of patients by place of residence</u>

2.5. Two peaks in call frequency were observed, a first peak from 9 to 11am and a second peak from 8 to 9pm, as shown in Figure 5.

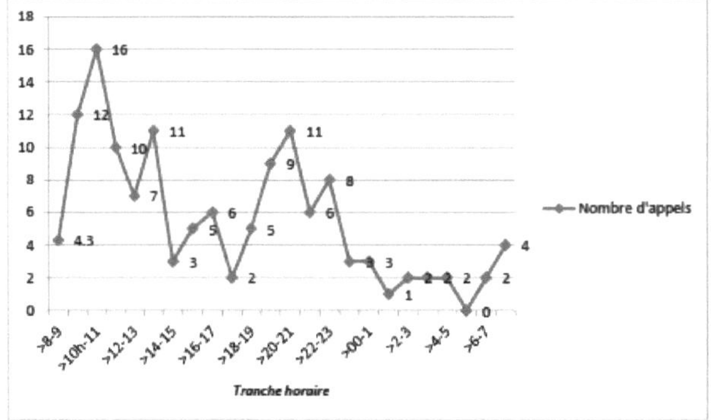

Figure 5: <u>Breakdown of patients by time of day</u>
2.5.<u>Call time according to activity time slots</u>

A study of the breakdown of calls by 4-hour working hours always shows a peak in activity from 8am to 12pm, with less activity from midday to midnight.
Activity was reduced (16%) between midnight and 8am.

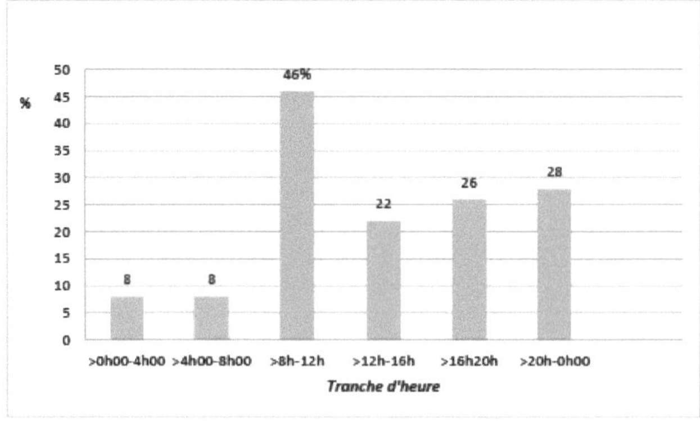

Figure 6: <u>Breakdown of calls by time of day</u>

3. Data from the telephone interview
3.1. Main reason for the phone call

Telephone questioning by the attending physician revealed a series of main reasons for calls, as detailed in Table III and Figure 7. Chest pain and dyspnea were the most frequent reasons for calling (60%).

Table III: <u>Main reason for call</u>

Design	Number of cases	%
Chest pain	54	26
Palpitations	13	6
Dyspnea	58	28
Neurological deficit	17	8
Altered state of consciousness	15	7
Drug intoxication	11	7
Change in general condition	12	5,5
Abdominal pain	11	5
Agitation, confusion	09	4
Fever	5	2,5
Other considerations	4	1,5
Total	**209**	**100 %**

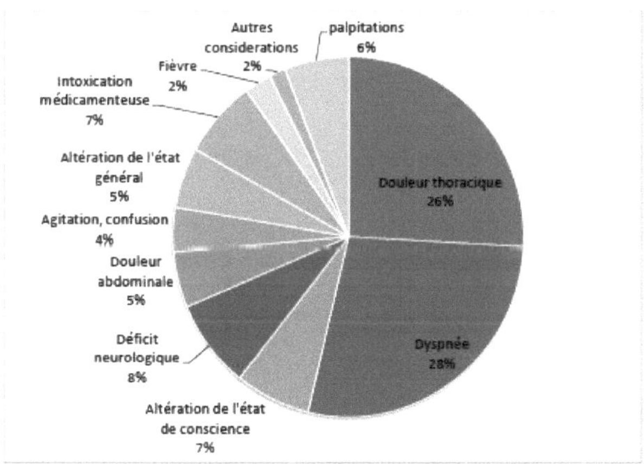

Figure 7: Main reason for the call

3.2. Patient history on appeal

In our study, 28% of patients had at least one cardiovascular risk factor. A cardiac antecedent was identified in 20% of patients and a respiratory antecedent in 28% of patients.

Table IV shows the various antecedents and pathologies identified by the regulating doctor via the telephone call.

Table IV: Patient history

	N =	%
Cardiovascular risk factors		
1. Diabetes	59	28
2. Smoking	45	21,5
3. HTA	41	19.5
4. Dyslipidemia	25	12
5. Sedentary or bedridden	22	10,5
Chronic bronchitis	47	22,5
Coronary artery bypass graft and/or stent holder	23	11
History of heart failure, valvulopathy	19	9
History of neoplasia, recent or current chemotherapy or radiotherapy	19	9
Psychiatric history	18	8,5
Previous or recent surgery	13	6
Asthmatic patients	11	5
Holder of an implantable defibrillator and/or pacemaker or mechanical valve	09	4
Oxygen therapy or NIV at home	05	2,5
History of pneumothorax	01	0,5

3.3. Clinical semiology

3.3.1. Typology and clinical features of on-call chest pain

In our study, 25% of patients had chest pain of an intriguing nature (a combination of several types). Chest tightness was present in 36% of cases. Retro-sternal burning was observed in 25% of cases (Table V).

Table V: Clinical features of chest pain on call

Types of pain	Number of cases	%
Chest tightness	24	36
Retro-sternal burn	17	25,5
Chest tingling	9	13,5
Stabbing pain	7	10
Pain suggestive of gastro- resophageal reflux disease	6	9
Posterior irradiation	4	6
Total	**67**	**100**
Poorly defined association or pain.	17	25

3.3.2. Clinical features of dyspnea on call

In our study, one patient in two (50%) had a position that improved respiratory gene. More than half the patients had expiratory dyspnoea associated with bronchial congestion and secretions (56%) (Table VI).

Table VI: Clinical features of dyspnea on call

Types of pain	Number of cases	%
Congestion with secretions	32	56
Dyspnea with wheezing	32	55,5
Dyspnea improved by a precise attitude or position	29	50
Expiratory dyspnea	28	48

	N=	%
Inspiratory dyspnea	11	19
Poorly expressed respiratory gene	08	13,5
High dyspnea		058,5

3.4. Treatment in progress

In our study, it was possible to identify the patient's current medical treatment in 75% of cases.

A quarter of patients were taking anti-platelet agents, and 21% were taking antihypertensive drugs (Table VII).

Table VII: <u>Current treatment of patients obtained by the regulatory physician</u>

Treatment in progress	N=	%
Treatment not precise - doesn't know his treatment	53	25,5
Antiplatelet agents	52	25
Antihypertensives	42	21,5
Beta 2 mimetic spray	34	16
Anticoagulants	28	13,5
Oral antidiabetics -insulin	18	8,5
Recent cessation of a treatment in progress	18	8,5
Psychiatric treatment	13	6,5
Recent addition of a new drug	12	6
The concept of a medication intake error	06	3

3.5. Suspected diagnosis by the attending physician

In our study, a cardiac origin was suspected in a third of cases (31%), and a respiratory pathology was suspected in 34%.

In 10% of cases, the attending physician was unable to identify a precise reason for the call (Table VIII).

Table VIII: <u>Diagnostic suspicions of the attending physician on call</u>

Suspected diagnosis by the regulatory physician	N=	%
Acute coronary syndrome (ACS)	42	20
COPD decompensation	32	15
Cerebrovascular Accident CVA	17	8
Respiratory infection: bronchopneumonia	16	8
Pulmonary embolism	15	7
Heart rhythm disorder	11	6
Nephritic colic	10	5
Psychiatric decompensation	10	5
acute lung syndrome	10	5
Asthma attacks	8	4
Convulsive seizure	7	3
Deliberate or accidental drug intoxication	5	2
Carbon monoxide (CO) poisoning	5	2
Other	21	10
Total	**209**	**100%**

3.6. Degree of prioritisation by the attending physician

A R1 priority exit with a doctor on board was initiated in one third of cases (Table IX).

Table IX: Degree of prioritisation of discharge by the attending physician

Category	Degree of urgency	Emergency level	N =	%
R1	Very urgent	Obvious or latent life-threatening emergency requiring the intervention of an emergency medical service.	67	32
R2	Urgent	Emergency requiring the dispatch of a local doctor, ambulance or VSAV within the agreed timeframe.	123	59
R3	Not urgent	Recourse to permanent care, as the delay is not a risk factor in itself.	19	9
R4	Not urgent	Medical advice.	0	0

3.7. Degree of diagnostic relevance assessed by the regulatory physician

In our study, the self-assessment of the degree of relevance of the diagnosis suspected by the attending physician (appendix 1) showed disparities.

In a third of cases, the suspicion was strong, and in a further 1/3 it was moderate (Figure 8).

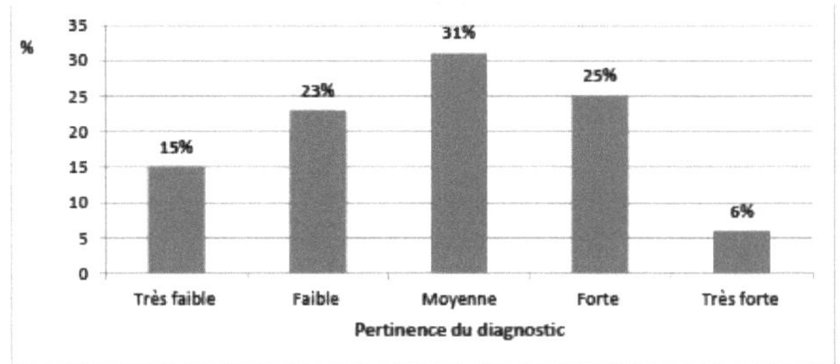

Figure 8: Degree of diagnostic relevance estimated by the medical regulator

4. Clinical characteristics of patients according to the operating physician

4.1. Suspected clinical diagnosis by the operating doctor

In our study, 22 patients were classified as non-urgent (10%), cardiac pathology was mentioned in 26.5% of cases and respiratory pathology in 33.5% (Table X).

Table X: Diagnostic suspicion of the intervention physician

Suspected diagnosis by the intervention doctor	N=	%
Acute coronary syndrome (ACS)	31	15
COPD decompensation	27	13
Respiratory infection: bronchopneumonia	24	11,5
Psychiatric decompensation, hysterical conversion	22	10
acute lung syndrome	18	8,5
Cerebrovascular Accident CVA	15	7
Pulmonary embolism	10	5
Asthma attacks	8	4
Parietal and osteoarticular pathology	8	4
Nephritic colic	7	3,5
Hypoglycaemic malaise	7	3,5
Heart rhythm disorder	6	3
Other	6	3
Deliberate or accidental drug intoxication	5	2,5

Carbon monoxide (CO) poisoning | 5 | 2,5
Trauma | 4 | 2
Convulsive seizure | 4 | 2
Total | 209 | 100%

4.2.CCMS classification of patients according to intervention physician

In our study, 93% of patients had a diagnostic or therapeutic procedure performed on site. In 5 cases (2.5%), a decision was made to limit care and active therapies (Table XI).

Table XI: <u>CCMS classification of patients at the time of surgery</u>

Class		N= %
Class 1	Stable patient requiring no diagnostic procedure or surveillance on the premises.	or2713
Class 2	Stable patient requiring at least one diagnostic procedure or or surveillance on the premises	2512
Class 3	Clinical condition which may worsen without firing vital prognosis	the10952
Class 4	Immediate vital or functional prognosis without need for life-saving treatment	2512
Class 5	Life-threatening with need for life support.	intervention2311
Class 6	Victim deceased before the arrival of the SMUR (no action resuscitation undertaken)	of00

4.3.Diagnostic suspicion of the interventional physician in the presence of chest pain

In our study, acute coronary syndrome was suspected in one out of two cases (46%). In 20% of cases, the chest pain was of parietal or psychiatric origin, leading to false emergencies (Table XII).**Table XII: <u>Diagnostic suspicion of the interventional physician in the presence of chest pain</u>**

Suspect diagnosis	Number of cases	%
Non-ST+ acute coronary syndrome (ACS) (+/- PAO)	22	33
ST+ acute coronary syndrome (with or without PAO)	9	13
Psychiatric pain	8	12
Pleuropneumonia /Pneumonia	8	12
Parietal pain	6	9
Pulmonary embolism	6	9
Heart rhythm disorder	6	9
Dissection of the aorta	2	3
Total	**67**	**100**

4.4.Diagnostic and therapeutic procedures carried out by the operating doctor

In our study, 3 out of 4 patients had their blood glucose measured by finger prick (79%) and their hemodynamic constants taken (85%). In more than half the cases, an ECG (64%), normobaric oxygen therapy (62%) and injectable medical treatment (56%) were initiated (Table XIII).

Table XIII: **Diagnostic and therapeutic procedures performed during the operation**

Suspect diagnosis	Number of	%
Hemodynamic monitoring	178	85
Finger glycemia	164	79
ECG	132	64
Normobaric oxygen therapy	128	62
Other injectable medical treatment	117	56
Analgesic treatment	78	37
NIV-CPAP	67	32
HbCO	35	16
Anti-ischemic treatment	31	15
Orotracheal intubation + mechanical ventilation	3	1

ECG: Electrocardiogram, **NIV**: Non-invasive ventilation, **CPAP**: Continuous positive airway pressure, **HbCO**: Carboxyhemoglobin.

5. Patient clinical data according to the emergency doctor

5.1. Degree of urgency in triage and patient management sector in the emergency department

In our study, 17% of patients were classified T1 on the Monastir triage scale and were admitted on arrival to the vital emergency department (SAUV) (Table XIV).

Table XIV: **Patient care sectors in emergency departments**

Care sector for patients with	Number of	%
USR (T2)	150	72
SAUV (T1, immediate emergency)	36	17
Medical-surgical consultation cubicle (T3, T4)	23	11
Total	**209**	**100**

SAUV: Secteur d'Accueil des Urgences Vital, **USR**: Unite de Surveillance Rappchee.

5.2. Additional examinations carried out in the emergency department

In our series, more than half the patients had an ECG (69%), a biological work-up (86%), a Troponin assay (57%), an arterial blood gas measurement (47%) and a chest X-ray (83%). CT or MRI imaging was requested in 25% of cases (Table XV).

Table XV: **Details of additional tests requested in emergency departments**

Further examination	Number of	%
Sampling, biological tests	180	86
Chest X-ray	175	83
ECG	145	69
Troponins	120	57
GDS	98	47
ProBNP	67	32
D-Dimeres	57	27
CT, MRI	52	25
Non-chest X-ray	48	23
ECBU	29	14
Lumbar puncture	14	7

ECG: Electrocardiogram, **GDS:** Blood gases, **ProBNP**: pro brain natriuretic peptide, **CT**: Computed tomography, **MRI:** Magnetic resonance imaging, **ECBU:** Cytobacteriological examination of urine.

5.3. Final etiological diagnosis according to the emergency doctor

In our series, cardiac pathology accounted for 11.5% of all emergency room diagnoses. Respiratory pathology represented 26% of cases, and in 27% of cases, the patient was classified as not very urgent and was seen in the medical-surgical consultation room (Table XVI).

Table XVI: <u>Etiological diagnosis confirmed in the emergency department</u>

Suspected diagnosis by the emergency doctor	N=	%
Psychiatric pathology, hysterical conversion	32	15
Parietal and osteoarticular pathology	26	12
COPD decompensation	24	11
Sepsis with a different starting point	20	9,5
Sepsis with respiratory onset	19	9
Cerebrovascular Accident CVA	13	6
(Acute lung tumour due to hypertensive peak	13	6
Other	9	4,5
Nephritic colic	9	4,5
Asthma attacks	8	4
Hypoglycemia	7	3,5
Heart rhythm disorder	6	3
Deliberate or accidental drug intoxication	5	2,5
Carbon monoxide (CO) poisoning	5	2,5
Acute coronary syndrome (ACS)	3	2,5
Pulmonary embolism	4	2
Convulsive seizure	4	2
Trauma	2	0,5
Total	**209**	**100%**

5.4. Referral and outcome of patients after emergency care

In our series, 44% of patients were kept in emergency for more than 48 hours. A third of patients (34%) were admitted to hospital. A return home was observed in 18% of cases (Table XVII).

Table XVII: <u>Referral of patients after emergency care</u>
emergency department

Patient referral	Number of cases	%	
Emergency hospitalisation > 48 hours	92	44	
Hospitalisation in a conventional ward	73		34
Leaving home without an inspection appointment	22	11	
Discharge home with outpatient appointment	15		7
Deaths		74	
Total209		**100**	

6. Analytical study

6.1. Comparison of the degree of patient prioritisation between the three doctors

In our study, there was a difference in the assessment of the "very high" and "very low" categories.

urgent" and "urgent" between the three doctors (Tables XVIII a,b,c, Figure 9.

Table XVIIIa: <u>Comparison of the degree of patient prioritisation between</u>

	MR, MI				
Emergency levels	Medical regulator		Intervention doctor		Degree of significance
Very urgent	R1	32%	CCMS 5.6	23%	2,05	p<0,01
Urgent	R2	59%	CCMS 3.4	64%	3,84	p >0,05
Not urgent	R3	09%	CCMS2	13%	6,21	p>0,05
Not urgent	R4	0%	CCMS1	0%		

Table XIXb: <u>Comparison of the degree of patient prioritisation between</u>

	MR, MU				
Emergency levels	Medical regulator		Emergency doctor		Degree of significance
Very urgent	R1	32%	T1	17%	2,41P<0,01
Urgent	R2	59%	T2	72%	1,78P<0,02
Not urgent	R3	09%	T3	11%	2,89P>0,05
Not urgent	R4	0%	T4	0%	-

Table XXc: <u>Comparison of the degree of patient prioritisation between</u>

	MI, MU				
Emergency levels	Doctor Intervention		Emergency doctor		Degree of significance
Very urgent	CCMS 5.6	23%	T1	17%	2,02 p> 0,05
Urgent	CCMS 3.4	64%	T2	72%	7,99 p>0,05
Not urgent	CCMS2	13%	T3	11%	3,54 p>0,05
Not urgent	CCMS1	0%	T4	0%	

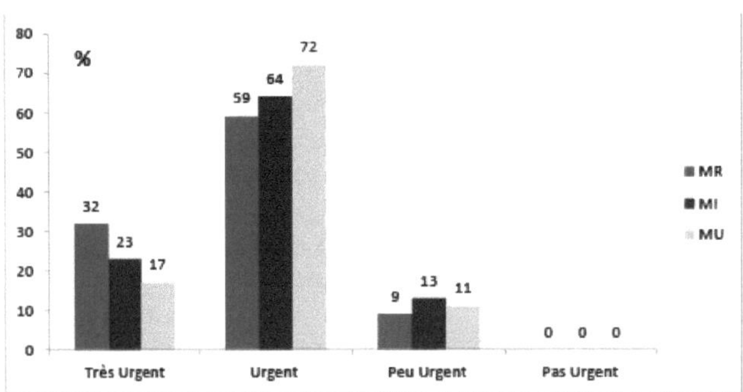

Figure 9: <u>Comparison of the degree of patient prioritisation between MR, MI and MU</u>

6.2. Diagnostic concordance

1.1.1. Comparison of the diagnosis suggested by the regulating doctor and the diagnosis suspected by the intervention doctor, by pathology

The difference was statistically significant for ACS, psychiatric pathology, parietal pathology (osteoarticular) and abdominal pathology (Table XIX).

Table XIX: <u>Comparison of suspected MR versus MI diagnosis by pathology</u>

Pathology group	MR(%)	MI(%)	Value of p

Pathology group			Value of p	
SCA	20	15	**0.003**	**DSS**
Psychiatric pathology	5	10	**0.035**	**DSS**
Parietal pathology	8	4	**0,028**	**DSS**
Abdominal pathology	20	14	**0,041**	**DSS**
Neurological pathology	11	9	2,37	DSNS
Respiratory pathology	27	28,5	1,28	DSNS
Cardiac pathology other than ACS	5	11,5	3,65	DSNS
Metabolic pathology, intoxications	4	8,5	2,87	DSNS
Other	5	5	**0,01**	**DSS**

SSD: Statistically significant difference. **NSSD**: Statistically non-significant difference.

1.2.Comparison of the diagnosis mentioned by the attending physician and the diagnosis confirmed by the emergency physician, by pathology

Table XX: <u>Comparison of suspected MR versus MU diagnosis by pathology</u>

Pathology group	MR(%)	MU(%)	Value of p	
SCA	20	2,5	**0,031**	**DSS**
Psychiatric pathology	5	15	**0,034**	**DSS**
Parietal pathology	8	12	**0,01**	**DSS**
Abdominal pathology	20	13,5	**0,001**	**DSS**
Neurological pathology	11	8	1,75	DSNS
Respiratory pathology	27	24	1,05	DSNS
Cardiac pathology other than ACS	5	11	**0,002**	**DSS**
Metabolic pathology, intoxications	4	7,5	2,89	DSNS
Other	5	6,5	3,02	DSNS

ACS: Acute Coronary Syndrome

6.3.Comparison of the diagnosis suspected by the emergency doctor and the diagnosis confirmed by the emergency doctor, by pathology

Table XXI: <u>Comparison of suspected MI versus MU diagnosis by pathology</u>

Pathology group	MI(%)	MU(%)	Value of p	
SCA	15	2,5	**0,01**	**DSS**
Psychiatric pathology	10	15	**0,05**	**DSS**
Parietal pathology	4	12	**0,02**	**DSS**
Abdominal pathology	14	13,5	1,038	DSNS
Neurological pathology	9	8	2,31	DSNS
Respiratory pathology	28,5	24	1,78	DSNS
Cardiac pathology other than ACS	11,5	11	2,75	DSNS
Metabolic pathology , poisoning	8,5	7,5	1,78	DSNS
Other	5	6,5	0,78	DSNS

SSD: Statistically significant difference. **NSSD**: Statistically non-significant difference.

7. Concordance of the etiological diagnosis between the regulatory physician and the intervention physician

Table XXI: <u>Characteristics of the Kappa coefficient of agreement MR Versus MI</u>

	Value	Standard error Asymptomatic	T Approximate	Meaning Approximate
Kappa	**7,681**	0,017	59,025	0,000

8. Consistency of diagnosis between the attending physician and the emergency physician

Table XXII: <u>Characteristics of the Kappa coefficient of agreement MR versus MU</u>

	Value	Standard error Asymptomatic	T Approximate	Meaning Approximate
Kappa	**7,012**	0,021	63,005	0,000

9. Concordance of the diagnosis between the emergency doctor and the operating doctor

Table XXIII: <u>Characteristics of the Kappa coefficient of concordance MI versus MU</u>

	Value	Standard error Asymptomatic	T Approximate	Meaning Approximate
Kappa	**8,203**	0,019	68,015	0,000

4 DATA ANALYSIS

Relevant results of the study

The concordance between the diagnosis suspected by the regulating doctor and that evoked by the intervention doctor was 0.768 and judged to be good.

The agreement between the diagnosis suspected by the attending physician and the emergency physician was 0.701 and considered good.

The concordance between the diagnosis evoked by the operating doctor and the emergency doctor was 0.820 and judged to be excellent.

The concordance was strong for the cardiac, respiratory, neurological and intoxication pathology groups. It was less consistent for psychiatric, parietal and digestive pathologies.

In the specific case of acute coronary syndrome, the diagnosis of ACS was suspected by the attending physician in 20% of cases of chest pain, and supported by the operating physician in 15% of cases. In emergency departments, the diagnosis of ACS was made in only 2.5% of cases.

Strengths and limitations of the study

Our study has both methodological and clinical relevance:

- Methodologically, the study was exhaustive, with few missing data (<10%), and the emergency room diagnosis used as a reference for the concordance study was obtained in 100% of cases, giving the statistical tests used a high level of power and our results a high degree of objectivity.

- In clinical terms, the study enabled a critical analysis of patient management procedures at the military SAMU/SMUR centre, identifying shortcomings and opening the door to new perspectives.

There were many limitations to our study, and hypothesis-confirmation bias cannot be totally ruled out in the absence of objective criteria for evaluating the clinical reasoning of pre-hospital doctors.

There were also selection biases due to the fact that the military SMUR centre essentially collaborates with a single emergency service and that the regulating doctors are themselves the intervention doctors, which could have influenced their clinical reasoning when carrying out this work.

It would be useful to carry out a study of situations where a medical team would have been required but was not sent to validate our results.

It was not possible to carry out a comparative study of the different SAMU military doctors according to their length of service, as all the SAMU military doctors were recruited at the same time.

The absence of national data in Tunisia on the operating mode of the various pre-hospital emergency centres prevented us from comparing our results at the local level, which would have enabled us to better assess the diagnostic and decision-making performance of our physicians.

Epidemiological data on the population studied

Age and gender

We collated 209 adult patients for whom a primary discharge was decided in the face of a medical pathology whose diagnosis was not obvious at the time of the call; this represents 33.5% of the activity of the military SAMU/SMUR for the year 2018. The remaining two-thirds of cases were discharges for traumatic or non-traumatic conditions with an obvious diagnosis, as well as secondary and paediatric discharges.

The mean age of the patients studied was 52 ±35 years, with a sex ratio of 2.21. In our study, 60% of patients were over 50 years of age and 33.5% were over 60 years of age. The advanced age of patients in our study was consistent with the literature.

In the Ben Arous Tunis SMUR study, the proportion of subjects aged over 60 was 31% [1]. These were patients treated for decompensations of a chronic cardiac or respiratory pathology.

Although our results are in line with the national [1,2] and international [3,4] literature concerning the age of patients, certain particularities are inherent to the organisation of health care in the Tunisian army:

- A proportion of young military patients are initially treated by the Advanced Medical Unit (AMU) doctor before calling the military SAMU/SMUR, which is considered to be a secondary transfer.

- A proportion of patients were transferred to emergency by the UMA's mobile unit, which constituted primary discharges not covered by the military SAMU/SMUR.

Both situations involved patients who did not meet the inclusion criteria for our study.

Table XXII details the average age and sex ratio of patients treated by different SAMU/SMUR centres:

Table XXIV: <u>Details of the average age and sex ratio of patients treated by different centres; SAMU/SMUR</u>

Author	SAMU/SMUR	N =	Average age (years)	Sex ratio	Remarks
Suberville[4]	Beaujon Paris	158	58 ± 18	0,16	
Melot[4]	Pontoise Paris	133	60	0,78	
Guille [3]	Nantes France	400	55 ± 20	0,6	
Mannai et al. [2]	SAMU 01 Tunis	87	59 ± 11	9	ST+ ACS
Ghazali et al. [1]	Ben Arous Tunis	193	57 years old	1.75	57 years old
Our study	Military Tunis	209	52 ± 35	2.21	

The predominance of men in our series is not a particularity of the SAMU/SMUR because the military population in Tunisia is essentially male. The sex ratio in a study by Mannai et al [2] (SAMU 01 of Tunis) on the management of ACS in the pre-hospital setting was 9.

Pathological background of patients

In our study, the elderly population was predominant, which explains the high rate of chronic pathologies compared with national rates in Tunisia. We found more chronic bronchitis sufferers, chronic heart failure sufferers and diabetics. Smoking in the military was well below the national average.

We cannot say that our sample was representative of the general Tunisian population. A statistical study should be carried out to confirm our hypotheses.

Table XXIII details the prevalence of the main pathologies found in the population studied and compares them with national averages:

Table XXV: <u>Details of the prevalence of the main diseases found in the population studied, compared with national averages</u>

Pathology	Prevalence in our study (%)	Tunisian national prevalence (%)
Smoking	21,5	50-60

HTA	19,5		30
Diabetes		28	19
Asthma	5		7,5
Heart failure	9		5,5
COPD	22,5		3,5

Socio-geographical data

The military SAMU/SMUR only provides care for people affiliated to the Tunisian army and their families. In our study, 42.5% of transferred patients were military pensioners, and 21% were family members of military personnel.

In our study, 86.5% of the population studied lived in Greater Tunis (the governorates of Tunis, Ariana, La Mannouba and Ben Arous). In 13.5% of cases, the military SAMU/SMUR was called upon to care for patients outside its area of activity on primary discharge for non-urgent medical conditions.

As part of its operational role, the military SAMU/SMUR coordinates and ensures the secondary transfer of patients who are victims of attacks or traffic accidents involving several victims. It covers the whole of Tunisia.

In the emergency department of the Tunis military hospital, transfers by the military SAMU/SMUR to the SAUV and USR sectors represented only 5% of the department's activity. This is explained by the fact that, despite regular information campaigns, the military medical aid centre remains little known among the military population: a large proportion of this population is unaware of the toll-free number, 199. Another proportion think that the military SAMU/SMUR is purely operational.

Profile of the pre-hospital doctor

Since its creation in 2013, the CMAMU has had its own pool of doctors. With a doctorate in medicine, they alternate between regulation and intervention activities. All the doctors assigned to the military SAMU/SMUR centre had more than 5 years' pre-hospital experience. This homogeneity in the profile of the doctors is a strong point in terms of the harmonisation of procedures and conduct and complementarity in patient care.

The same profile of doctors was found in the SAMU/SMUR of Marrakech: all the responders were general practitioners with competence in emergency medicine [5]. Omri et al [6] in their study carried out at the SAMU 03 of Sousse and concerning the study of pre-hospital diagnostic omissions in a traumatic context, 89% of the discharges were carried out by residents or interns in training.

Within the SAMU 01 of Tunis, pre-hospital discharges are carried out by a heterogeneous population of general practitioners, residents in training and university graduates specialising in emergency medicine and temporary doctors.

In Ribe's study [7], the regulating doctor was a general practitioner in 64.4% of cases, and an assistant in 33%. In 2.6% of cases, it was an associate.

In a study of practices at France's Centre 15, Giroud noted that the involvement of GPs in medical regulation is an undeniable success. The complementarity between GPs and emergency doctors guarantees a coordinated, effective and appropriate response to the growing diversity of emergency calls. The work of GPs enables the development of medical advice and the limitation of home visits [8].

Medical regulation

Medical regulation is a medical procedure carried out over the telephone (or by any other telecommunication device) by a regulating doctor. The medical act is a medical decision that involves the individual responsibility of the doctor. This decision is based on all the information available to the doctor, and its aim is to determine and activate the appropriate medical response for each situation as quickly as possible [9].

Medical records

The recommendations of the French haute autorite de sante (HAS) published in 2012 stipulate that [9 -12] :

- Any call concerning a patient received at the medical regulation centre leads to the opening of a medical regulation file. A summary of the computerised medical file used to support medical regulation will be included in the personal medical file (DMP) when it becomes operational.

- The file is only closed once we have been assured that the patient's care has been relayed or completed.

At the military SAMU/SMUR, patients' medical files are only closed once they have been discharged from hospital. Monitoring continues during the patient's stay in the emergency department and during their admission to a conventional hospital ward. When the patient is discharged, the DMP is closed.

In our study, the files were 100% usable because of the double archiving of the files (paper and digital versions) and the daily evaluation of the transfer forms before archiving.

The work by Mtiraoui A. et al. (2017) [13], the aim of which was to assess the quality of keeping and filling in the regulation and intervention file within the SMUR 05 of Gabes, showed an overall rate of non-compliance of the intervention file (missing data) of 40% due to a heterogeneity of practices and the absence of systematic feedback on the DMPs.

Early call-back procedures, more or less at a distance from the call, targeting situations at risk for the patient, are an interesting alternative when it is impossible to obtain information concerning the management of patients transferred to emergency or during their hospitalisation. At the SAMU/SMUR in Nantes, the call-back rate observed in a study of outgoing calls was 45%, and the rate of corrective second medical regulation was less than 2%. More than nine times out of ten, a protocolised management of the callback by the MRA was sufficient [7,13].

Time of call

In our study, two peaks in call frequency were observed, a first peak from 8am to 12pm and a second peak from 8pm to midnight. The same findings have been reported in the literature.

Kandri Z. [5] specified that 72% of the activities of the SAMU/SMUR of Marrakech took place between 8 and 20h. In Ribe's study at the SAMU/SMUR in Nantes [7], 79% of activity was also between 8 and 20 hours, with a peak between 8 and 12 hours.

Penverne et al [14], in a study of the performance indicators of the Nantes 15 centre, came to the same conclusions as our study: two peaks in frequency from 8 to 12 am and from 8 pm to midnight.

These two comparative curves show call frequencies as a function of time (Figure 10).

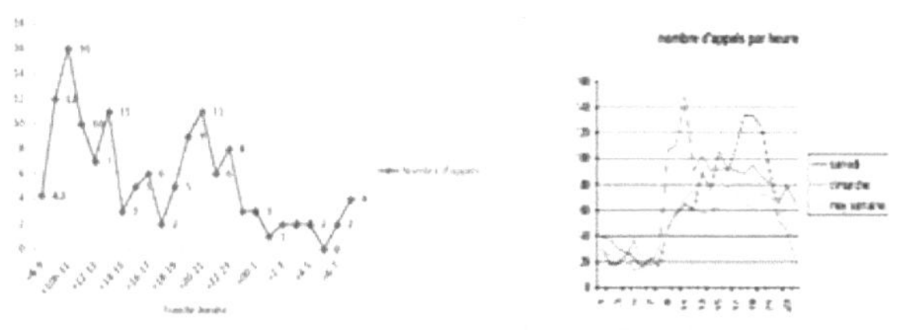

Figure 10: <u>Call frequencies by time of day</u>

Reason for call

In our study, cardiorespiratory pathology accounted for 68% of the reasons for call. These were decompensation of chronic pathologies in 89% of cases; acute lung disease, ischemic pathology, decompensation of chronic obstructive pulmonary disease. Chest pain represented 32% of the reasons for call, and dyspnea was present in 26% of cases.

Our findings are consistent with those in the literature. Cardiovascular pathology is over-represented in all the studies (55 to 72%), essentially represented by ischemic heart disease: unstable angina in almost 40.5% of cases, acute myocardial infarction, also acute pulmonary rearrhythmia, cardio-genic shock and cardiorespiratory arrest of suspected or confirmed cardiovascular origin [5, 7, 8, 10, 14, 17, 18].

In a large proportion of the literature, traumatic pathology outranked the cardiorespiratory pathology group. However, in our study, traumatic pathology was one of the non-inclusion criteria. The elimination of the traumatic pathology group from these studies is consistent with the general findings of the literature.

Performance indicators for an emergency medical service

The efficiency of an emergency system is measured by its ability to provide the right service in the right place at the right time [12]. Several factors can influence the quality of pre-hospital patient care, such as the geographical distribution and frequency of calls, the number of resources, staff skills, the quality of equipment and vehicles, the location of hospitals, the location of bases, and the adequacy of organisation and communications [11,12].

Our study is part of a quality initiative launched in 2017 by the military emergency medical assistance centre to obtain certification for the military SAMU/SMUR.

The evaluation of emergency medical services is based on a dual assessment:

- Appreciation of quantitative parameters: well-defined in the literature
- Appreciation of qualitative parameters: genuine indicators of a service's performance in relation to the quality of the medical decision that are less well 48
defined.

Quantitative assessment parameters

There are several performance indicators which are naturally linked to the organisational, logistical and human issues of EMS/Remote Medical Services systems. Thus, there are three main categories of performance measures used in the literature [5, 11, 12, 19]:

Time indicators

They involve a series of delays and times, and few studies have looked at patient management times. In Tunisia, only one study has been published on pre-hospital patient management times: in the study by Ghazali et al [1], the mean medicalisation time was 52 ± 21 minutes and the mean intervention time was 79 ± 38 minutes. Several indicators of time

23

and delay have been identified in the literature [11,19]:
- Average response rate
- Tripping time
- Waiting time
- Coverage rate within T
- Non-coverage rate
- Treatment access time
- Service time-Waiting time
- Queue size - percentage of non-response
- Distance travelled

Survival rate indicators

They define the percentage of patients who survive an accident during a given period (e.g. after accident report, before final care, after admission to a care facility). Although this is a measure of quality of care that reflects the ability of an emergency medical service to respond adequately to its primary objective of saving lives [19], very little literature has been devoted to it because of the difficulty of linking precise quantitative measures of survival rates to organisational changes in the care process.

Cost indicators

The financial aspect is rarely taken into account when evaluating the performance of a pre-hospital medical service, and includes investment and operating costs. In the literature, few studies have looked at this aspect of evaluation [11,12], although it is relevant to carry out a cost-effectiveness analysis by comparing the costs of each alternative with the time saved or the improvement in survival rate obtained that is necessary to achieve the expected objective at the lowest cost.

Qualitative assessment parameters

The aim of these indicators is to assess the match between the care offered and the patient's actual needs [3, 7, 14]. Their evaluation should help, among other things, to identify the shortcomings and dysfunctions of a facility that can be improved (internal evaluation), and to improve the overall care of patients.

It should also facilitate comparison with the activity of identical structures (regional or even national).

Several criteria must be taken into account to assess this performance: pre-hospital diagnosis, assessment of the patient's clinical severity, the care load required and the patient's immediate outcome [3, 7, 14]. These quality indices help to distinguish the four main levels of performance of a pre-hospital medical service.

Diagnostic performance

There are a number of advantages to comparing diagnoses made for the same patients, in outpatient departments, pre-hospital departments and then in hospital reception departments (emergency departments or other departments):

- Facilitate the identification of avoidable diagnostic errors, which are a source of alteration in therapeutic management and therefore of increased patient morbidity and mortality.

- Facilitate the identification of inappropriate care pathways used by patients. - The comparison of suspected diagnoses (after medical regulation, and after treatment by the SMUR) with reference diagnoses (receiving hospital services) [8, 11, 16, 20]. This is facilitated by the common use of a single classification used to code pathologies.

Decision-making performance

It corresponds to the match between the response provided and the patient's actual need for care [7]. It is based, in part, on an assessment of the clinical severity of the patient treated in the pre-hospital and emergency departments.

She appreciates it:

- Justifying or not justifying the resources committed to a patient
- Decisional deficiencies, represented by patients (benefiting from medical regulation) admitted to emergency departments in a state of vital distress without prior medical treatment.

Analysis of these 'atypical trajectories' should help to reduce the number of admissions to emergency departments by improving patient referrals.

Therapeutic performance

It corresponds to the therapeutic delay [17]: the time taken to activate an emergency medical service and the time taken for the emergency medical service to intervene. These times are of vital importance in the management of certain pathologies. Longer response times lead to increased patient morbidity and mortality (thrombolysis in acute myocardial infarction, early administration of antibiotics in purpura fulminans, etc.). Therapeutic performance will depend on shortening these delays.

Technical performance

It corresponds on the one hand to the resources made available to the SAMU (telephony, teletransmission, database) and the SMUR (ECG transmission, resuscitation equipment, therapeutics), and on the other hand to the care load deployed during SMUR interventions. Assessment of this care load in the emergency medical services (which is closely correlated with the clinical severity of patients in the majority of cases) must be based on the use of measurement tools that are relevant, simple, quick to use, objective and adapted to the pre-hospital context.

Decision-making performance: Degree of prioritisation

Call prioritisation

For regulating physicians, analysis of the performance indicators of a regulation centre must necessarily take into account the level of call prioritisation [16].

The classification of degrees of urgency in regulation, established by the SAMU de France in 2004, revised in 2009 and in 2016, was the one adopted by the centre militaire d'aide medicale urgente since its creation in 2014, and distinguishes 4 levels of urgency for the decisions of the regulating doctor (Appendix 4).

In our study, 32% of calls were classified as "very urgent" (R1) with a life-threatening outcome, and 59% of calls were classified as "urgent" (R2). Our results are consistent with the literature. Three franchised studies reported virtually the same figures. No Tunisian publication on call prioritisation was found in our literature review (Table XXIV).

Table XXVI: Comparison of the different studies carried out in terms of call priorities

Author	SAMU	of exits R1	of exits R2	Total R1+R2
Ribe, 2015 [7]	Nantes, France	37	50	87%
Rettori, 2013 [4]	Arles, France	26	40	66%
Buttes, 2004 [3]	Nantes, France	14	64	78%
Our study, 2018	CMAMU, Tunisia	32	59	91%

Catego risation during surgery

The advantage of the classifications produced by the emergency doctor, also known as the effector, is that they categorise the populations of patients treated by the emergency medical services into groups of homogenous clinical severity, each reflecting different medical management strategies.

The use of a single classification method (or comparable classifications) would have two advantages:

- Epidemiological: this would enable a qualitative assessment of the activity of a SMUR and facilitate inter-hospital comparisons.

- Economic: it could be an important factor in the procedures for accrediting a SMUR by helping to quantify the budget allocations and human resource requirements necessary for its operation.

The indirect result would therefore be an improvement in the quality of care provided to pre-hospital patients.

We found two relevant classifications in the literature, both derived from the Clinical Classification of Emergency Illness (CCED):

- The modified CCMU classification: CCMUm, valid only at regional level in France in the Midi-Pyrenees region (Appendix 6).

- The clinical classification of SMUR patients: CCMS, developed and validated nationally in France during multicentre studies [3, 7] (Appendix 5).

In the Gille des Buttes study [3], the aim of which was to verify the concordance of these two classifications, both inspired by the same "parent" classification: the CCMU, despite a few differences, the concordance of the CCMUm and the CCMS appeared to be excellent, with high concordance (Kappa coefficient = 0.93).

In our study, we chose to use the CCMS classification. For 86% of patients in the sample (cumulative percentages of classes 3, 4, 5 and 6 respectively), pre-hospital medicalisation was justified because the patient was judged to be at least likely to become clinically worse. For 13% of patients (the combined percentages for CCMS classes 1 and 2 respectively), pre-hospital medicalisation was theoretically unjustified, as it concerned stable patients requiring a general medical examination or non-medical transport. In reality, it was more often than not a case of potentially serious pathologies on call, warranting a clinical examination or at least a hemodynamic assessment and a finger-stick blood glucose test, which was ultimately reassuring. In the majority of cases, therefore, the resources employed did not appear to be unjustified.

In the literature, we have observed the same trend in the distribution of patients into classes using the CCMS or CCMUm classification; a majority of patients classified as categories 3, 4 and 5 and few patients classified as categories 1 and 2 on the two scales [7, 16].

In our series, the diagnostic procedures most frequently performed as the minimum initial work-up were hemodynamic monitoring in 85% of cases, GAD in 79% of cases and ECG in 64% of cases.

With regard to the therapies used in the field, normobaric oxygen therapy was initiated in 62% of cases. NIV was used in 32% of cases. In the case of acute coronary syndromes with ST-segment elevation, anti-ischemic therapy was initiated in all cases, but no thrombolysis was performed, since the ST+ protocol at the military hospital recommends primary angioplasty, which is available 24 hours a day.

Emergency triage

Several triage scales have been validated and applied in emergency departments. In our study, we opted for the Monastir Triage Scale (Appendix 7) adopted by the emergency department of the Tunis military hospital, where 100% of the patients in the study were admitted.

In our study, 17% of patients transferred via the military SAMU/SMUR were admitted to the SAUV, 72% to the USR and only 11% of patients were examined in a medicosurgical consultation room.

Two confounding biases can be advanced here concerning the relevance of patient admission to the SAUV and USR sectors:

-    Sometimes, due to a lack of space in the SAUV, the patient was admitted to the USR.

-    In the absence of a UHCD in the emergency department of the Tunis military hospital, patients are frequently admitted to the USR.

Comparison of the assessment of patients' clinical severity

In our study, there was a statistically significant difference in the degree of prioritisation and therefore in the estimation of severity between the three doctors for the 'very urgent' and 'urgent' categories.

There was no statistically significant difference between patients classified as non-urgent and urgent. There was good agreement between the three doctors in identifying non-urgent patients.

There is a tendency for the regulating doctor to overestimate the seriousness of the case, which can be explained by :

-    The lack of resources to objectively assess the patient's condition compared with the resources available to the emergency doctor or the doctor on call.

-    Fear and lack of confidence alienate the caller, who in turn tends to exaggerate the symptomatology.

Danet et al [21] explained that this phenomenon of exaggeration is due to the user's subjectivity, which prevails over their a priori categorisation within a framework.

In fact, "healthcare professionals complained that they were the victims of a utilitarian use of emergency care by patients, who abused this technical tool in a logic of free and excessive consumption".

Matuszak [15], in his study, even reports that callers are increasingly demanding in terms of the urgency of their request, thus influencing the objectivity of the regulating doctor. For example, a minor finger injury becomes insurmountable without the intervention of a team of two or three people, to reassure everyone and avoid the risk of liability. An anxiety attack ("tetany", "spasmophilia") can end up on an emergency gurney, because there's not enough time or consideration to defuse it on the spot. So how do you navigate between medical responsibility and ambulance abuse, and the ever-increasing demands for access to these services?

A second argument put forward by Danet [21], in the same study, is that the precariousness of a large number of residents who cannot find a response in their immediate environment (no access to transport to get to hospital, no financial means to see a GP) forces them to contact pre-hospital services.

-    Intuition; despite the existence of decision-making algorithms, regulators tend to trust their intuition more than the algorithms.

In a study by Brunel et al [22], the aim was to compare the diagnostic performance of the calculated probability algorithm for non-ST+ ACS versus the intuitive probability. The Youden index was 0.30 for the algorithm's calculated probability (sensitivity 68%, 95% CI [52-80%] and for specificity 62%, 95% CI [56-67%]) and 0.43 for clinical intuition (sensitivity 50%,

95% CI [3565%] and specificity 93%, 95% CI [89-95%]). The author concluded that the intuition of the emergency physician in the EMS department has better specificity than the calculated probability algorithm for diagnosing high-risk non-ST+ ACS.

In our study, the management of ACS represented a situation in which the overestimation of pre-hospital doctors played a major role. ACS was suspected by the attending physician in 20% of cases of chest pain, and in 15% of cases the diagnosis of ACS was retained by the interventional physician. In only 2.5% of cases was the diagnosis confirmed in the emergency department.

Diagnostic performance: Concordance study
Overall performance

In our study :

- The degree of agreement between the diagnosis suspected by the attending physician and that of the emergency physician was good (kappa =0.70).
- Agreement between the diagnoses of the interventional physician and the emergency physician was excellent (kappa = 0.82).

We found a high degree of concordance between the pre-hospital diagnosis and that of the emergency department. Overall, our results were better than those found in the literature.

In the French study by Senicourt (2016) [22], the diagnostic concordance between prehospital and emergency departments was K= 0.687. After including partially concordant diagnoses, the Kappa coefficient reached 0.728. The study by Romain (2012) put the concordance rate at 0.662 for diagnoses that were 100% concordant [14].

In 2003, Poiner et al [17] carried out an American study evaluating the degree of agreement between the pre-hospital diagnosis of paramedics and that of the emergency department for cardiac dyspnoea. The kappa index was 0.60, 95% CI [0.51-0.69], for dyspnea of respiratory origin, the kappa index was 0.69, 95% CI [0.59, 0.79].

When the diagnosis was consistent with simultaneous cardiac and respiratory decompensation (n=24), responders treated 7 patients as having cardiac decompensation and 13 patients as having respiratory decompensation. Only four patients were correctly treated pre-hospital for both cardiac and respiratory pathologies [17].

Several factors come into play to explain the high concordance in our series:

- **Working procedures**

The SAMU/SMUR military centre is equipped with decision-making procedures and algorithms, valid within the regulation, as well as the existence of algorithms and technical intervention sheets valid within the framework of the centre's certification project.

There is close collaboration with the military hospital's emergency department on working procedures and the establishment of anticipation and preparation protocols.

The SAMU/SMUR military centre and the emergency service were heavily involved in drawing up the military hospital's white plan, and are represented on the steering committee for the action strategy in the event of a mass influx of injured people.

- **Characteristics of doctors**

All the doctors working at the military SAMU/SMUR centre have been trained in call taking, decision making and pre-hospital medicine. These are the same doctors who are alternately assigned to regulation or intervention.

- The uniformity of practices is due, among other things, to the fact that all the doctors working at the military emergency medical aid centre have the same profile. The centre does not have a team of temporary doctors or doctors in training (residents or interns).

Few studies in Tunisia have focused on the characteristics of physicians practising in the pre-hospital setting. In the study by Omri et al [6] (2017) at SAMU 03 in Sousse, on the study of diagnostic omissions in pre-hospital care in a traumatic context, the diagnostic discordance was 25.5%, judged high by the author with a vital prognosis at stake in 29% of cases. In the same study, 89% of discharges were carried out by residents or interns in training.

- **Feedback and retroaction: medical relevance**

The value of feedback and feedback of information about patient diagnosis and patient outcome plays an essential role in improving the medical appropriateness of pre-hospital emergency departments.

The medical relevance of the act of regulation is assessed solely on the basis of the information acquired during the telephone interview. However, information acquired subsequently is useful in understanding the case. It would be important to know the diagnosis made during the subsequent management of the case in order to inform the team's reflections on the practice of medical regulation. Feedback to the regulating doctor is currently very incomplete [8,22]. It generally only concerns the most serious cases, and only at the earliest stages of their management.

In France, feedback to the department takes the form of more or less systematic letters (reports from receiving departments), targeted messages (generally complaints) or registers (coronary syndromes, strokes, head injuries, etc.) [23]. Feedback to the attending physician is not always recorded and shared within the department. Conversely, it is not easy for the department to send information received at a distance from the act of medical regulation to each of the professionals concerned. Assessing medical appropriateness requires management of this feedback; this applies to all cases, not just the most serious [22, 25,26]. Within the military centre, a number of strengths were highlighted:

- Daily group debriefing of all outings.

- Continuous feedback from patients after admission to the emergency department and hospitalisation in an appropriate department, right through to discharge from hospital. The DMP is not closed until the patient leaves hospital.

- The existence of a database covering all patients with chronic pathologies who are likely to return to hospital fairly frequently. Knowing patients' antecedents before they are discharged enables them to be anticipated and better managed during the operation.

- **Continuing medical education (DPC)**

- as part of the centre's certification process, medical training has been developed over the last few years, with the appointment of a quality referral doctor responsible for monitoring training courses.

- Simulation training based on fictitious scenarios or real-life situations is common practice at the SAMU/SMUR military centre. The military SAMU/SMUR has an emergency care teaching centre (CESU), located within the hospital itself. Simulation training in emergency procedures and resuscitation is available for doctors, paramedics and nurses working at the centre.

The North American study by Jonathan et al [27] simultaneously assessed cognitive knowledge and simulated field performance. The results showed a strong association between field performance and the cognitive knowledge of a pre-hospital responder assessed during a simulation exercise of a real intervention case.

Performance by disease group

Pathological groups with poor diagnostic concordance

It appears that certain groups of specific pathologies do not provide a high level of concordance, probably because these groups are not so specific. The "parietal pathology" group, which includes all non-traumatic osteo-articular and musculo-ligamentary pathology, and the "other medical" pathology group most often include imprecise and poorly systematised diagnoses in the face of an unfamiliar picture for the regulating physician or the physician performing the operation. On the other hand, after hospitalisation, the main diagnosis will generally be more precise.

Abdominal pathology is also a speciality prone to discordance. Most frequently, an abdominal syndrome evoked on call leads the attending physician to suspect a cardiovascular pathology (inferior MI, ruptured abdominal aortic aneurysm, etc.). The final diagnosis will be made by the operating doctor or, better still, by the hospital doctor, on the basis of clinical and paraclinical examinations.

Psychiatric pathology represents the medical group where the discordance was quite strong, and the regulating doctor tends to overestimate the psychiatric problem, even if it is a hysterical conversion crisis. Secondly, on the assumption that all psychiatric pathology is organic in origin until proven otherwise, the pre-hospital doctor finds himself obliged to transfer the patient to an emergency facility.

Pathological groups with high diagnostic concordance

In our study, the concordance was strong for the cardiac, respiratory, neurological and intoxication pathology groups.

We found that the strong concordance in the cardiac and respiratory groups concerned only chronic pathologies. Since ACS is an acute event, there was a high degree of discordance, based on the principle that all chest pain is ACS until proven otherwise.

For neurological pathologies, the concordance was strong only for acute events (stroke, sudden motor deficit, convulsion), for example MR=8 versus MI=7 and MU=6 for stroke and MR=3 versus MI=2 and MU=2 for convulsions, as well as episodes of acute intoxication.

In the case of deliberate drug intoxication (VDI), most doctors were conflicted as to the suspected ingested product, despite the existence of decision-making algorithms based on toxidromes.

The study by Morisson et al [8] concluded that the regulating physician frequently opted for a lesser choice in terms of medical treatment, but in all cases, the regulating physician mainly referred patients to emergency services rather than to a specialised poison control centre.

Outlook

- The results of our study have helped, even if only partially, to highlight the problem of harmonising practices within the various pre-hospital emergency centres. We found a great deal of variability in practices and evaluation methods. The lack of local Tunisian data prevented a clearer assessment of pre-hospital practices in Tunisia.

Harmonising practices between pre-hospital and hospital emergency services will provide solutions to the problem of recurrent saturation of emergency services. We recommend setting up care networks organised around pre-hospital medicine. This approach would bring multiple benefits;

• Reducing overcrowding in emergency departments

• Reduce the healthcare costs generated by "unnecessary" visits to emergency departments and the time it takes to treat certain patients by favouring dedicated short circuits.

In Tunisia, according to the national health institute, the rate of elderly people receiving pre-hospital care is set to increase in the coming years as a result of the ageing of the population. In 2019, the proportion of people aged over 60 was 13%, rising to 20.1% by

2039 [28].

Implementing a proactive strategy within pre-hospital services and emergency departments for the care of the elderly (adapted organisational and logistical procedures) is more than necessary these days.

The use of telemedicine to diagnose and prioritise pre-hospital patients is an excellent alternative that several learned societies and authors encourage [2, 7, 9, 10]. Its aim is to improve pre-hospital management times and consequently the performance indices of a SAMU/SMUR service. Giraud et al [25] even suggest that a telemedicine-equipped medical regulation centre can organise a network of consultants around it who can provide specialist advice in certain specific cases and establish a network of complementarity between the various pre-hospital and hospital emergency services on a local and regional scale.

In a study by Rasmussen et al [29] in Denmark, telemedicine was used to confirm STEMI in 84% of cases, enabling patients to be transferred directly to an interventional cardiology laboratory for primary angioplasty. In the same study, telemedicine shortened transfer times to less than 90 minutes from the first medical contact within a radius of 75 km.

Using simulation to develop regulation and intervention scenarios helps to improve the performance indicators of a pre-hospital medical service. Simulation is particularly useful in mass influx situations and for managing multiple casualty situations.

Implementing feedback and retroaction procedures, or structuring new procedures for monitoring patients in the immediate and medium term, is a necessary step in improving pre-hospital practices [8].

5 Conclusions

Saving a patient's life, stabilising their condition and providing appropriate referral are the cornerstones of pre-hospital emergency medicine. Faced with this challenge, in a very short space of time and in conditions that are often unexpected and sometimes dangerous, the emergency doctor practising in the pre-hospital setting must provide a high level of decision-making, technical, diagnostic and therapeutic performance in the face of extremely varied medical and surgical pathologies.

The aim of our study was to evaluate the diagnostic performance of the Tunis military emergency medical aid centre (CMAMU) by comparing the diagnosis made by the regulating doctor on call and the intervention doctor at the scene with the confirmatory diagnosis made at the reference emergency department. The diagnostic performance of the military emergency medical assistance centre was judged by comparing the diagnosis made in the pre-hospital setting by the regulating and intervention doctors with that made by the reference emergency doctor (the main assessment criterion of our study). Decision-making performance was assessed by evaluating the degree to which patients were prioritised according to clinical severity (secondary assessment criterion in our study).

We recorded 209 primary discharges with a non-obvious diagnosis in 2018, representing 34% of the centre's overall activity.

The mean age of the patients included in our study was 51.2 ± 35 years, with a sex ratio of 2.21. Older subjects (over 60 years of age) represented 31% of the study population.

With regard to the social profile of the population studied, 94% of patients were members of the Tunisian army (active or retired) and 86.5% lived in Greater Tunis.

Regulation and intervention activities at the military emergency medical aid centre were carried out 100% by the centre's doctors, who had more than 5 years' experience in pre-hospital medicine.

An analysis of the times when the military SMUR was called out showed two peaks in daily activity: from 8am to 12pm and from 8pm to midnight.

The main reason for the call was cardiac or respiratory pathology in 68% of cases, with chest pain and dyspnoea at the top of the list.

A priority medical discharge classified as R1 and R2 by the regulating doctor was initiated in 91% of cases.

A diagnostic or therapeutic procedure was undertaken at the scene in 87% of cases. In 23% of cases, the patient's vital prognosis was at risk on arrival (CCMS 4 and 5), and in 2.5% of cases, a decision was made to limit or stop active treatment (LATA).

In 100% of cases, the patient was transferred to the emergency department of the Tunis military hospital, the patient was admitted to the SAUV in 17% of cases and to the USR in 72% of cases.

In our series, 44% of patients were kept in emergency for a period of 48 hours. 34% of patients were admitted to hospital. A return home was decided in 18% of cases.

Two pathological groups predominated in SMUR discharges (60%): cardiovascular pathology (32%), mainly represented by chest pain, and respiratory pathology (28%), led by dyspnea.

In our study, re-evaluation of the clinical severity of patients and therefore of the degree of prioritisation of management by the regulating doctor (degree of absolute or relative urgency) by the intervention doctor (CCMS score) compared with that of the emergency doctor (triage score) showed a statistically significant discrepancy which only concerned patients with a high level of urgency ("very urgent" and "urgent") due to over-estimation by pre-hospital doctors.

Critical analysis of the diagnostic concordance between pre-hospital doctors and hospital doctors showed strong concordance for cardiovascular and respiratory pathologies. On the other hand, agreement was poor for parietal and psychiatric pathologies, in line with the principle of always ruling out an organic cause before considering a psychiatric one.

In the specific case of acute coronary syndrome, the diagnostic concordance between the three doctors was low (20% and 15% in pre-hospital care compared with 2.5% in the emergency department).

Because of the originality of the work, our study was doubly relevant:

- Methodological relevance: an exhaustive series of all the cases treated by the military SMUR centre, with few missing data and complete patient traceability.

- Clinical relevance: our study highlighted the high quality of patient care provided by the military SAMU/SMUR.

Despite the efforts made by the CMAMU to ensure optimum care for patients entitled to treatment, the harmonisation of practices within the various pre-hospital emergency centres remains a problem that needs to be resolved in the near future.

The introduction of a proactive strategy in pre-hospital services and emergency departments for the care of the elderly is more than necessary these days.

And the use of telemedicine to diagnose and prioritise pre-hospital patients represents an excellent alternative for boosting the performance of our pre-hospital care services and the subsequent management of our patients.

6 REFERENCES

1. Ghazali H, Souissi S, Touj H, Chermiti I, Ben Soltane I, Chaieb I, et al. Evaluation of the workload of a mobile emergency and resuscitation service during primary discharges. Evaluation et pre-hospitalier. Ann Fr Med Urgence. 2019;(7):5.

2. Manai H, Zelfani S, Aloui A, Yedes A, Zamiti A, Daghfous M, et al. Coronary syndromes with persistent ST-segment elevation in the pre-hospital setting: factors predictive of mortality. Evaluation et pre-hospitalier. Ann Fr Med Urgence. 2019;(1):18.

3. Gille des Buttes. Evaluation de la gravite des patients pris en charge au service medical d'urgence et de reanimation: comparaison de deux classifications: la CCMS et la CCMU modifiee [These]. Medecine: Nantes; 2004. 58p.

4. Suberville M, Belpomme V, Lenglet H, Casalino E. Enquete de satisfaction en prehospitalier [online]. Soc Fr Med Urgence. [cited 05/07/2013]; [about 1 screen]. Disponible a I'URL :
https://www.sfmu.org/upload/70 formation/02 eformation/02 congres/Urgences/urgences2013/donnees/communications/resume/posters/CP225.pdf.

5. Kandri Z. Le service medical d'urgence et de reanimation primaire: bilan du service d'aide medicale urgente regional de Marrakech et perspectives de développement [These]. Medecine: Marrakech; 2015. 115p.

6. Omri M, Bouaouina H, Kraiem H, Chebili N, Methamem M, Jaouadi MA, et al. Lesions oubliees chez les traumatises en pre-hospitalier. Tunis Med. 2017;95(5):336-40.

7. Ribe N. Evaluation de la performance diagnostique au service d'aide medicale urgente/service medical d'urgence et de reanimation de Nantes [These]. Medicine: Nantes; 2005. 111p.

8. Morrison L, Cassidy L, Welsford M. Clinical performance feedback to paramedics: what they receive and what they need. Acad Emerg Med. 2017;1(2):87-97.

9. Haute Autorite de Sante. Modalites de prise en charge d'un appel de demande de soins non programmes dans le cadre de la regulation medicale [Online]. Haute Autorite de Sante, [cited 01/03/2011];[about 1 screen]. Available at URL: https://www.has-sante.fr/jcmsZc 1061039/en/modalites- de-prise-en-charge-d-un-appel-de-demande-de-soins-non-programmes- dans-le-cadre-de-la-regulation-medicale.

10. Haute Autorite de Sante. Prise en charge de I'infarctus du myocarde a la phase aiguë en dehors des services de cardiologie [On line]. Haute Autorite de Sante, [cited 27/04/2007];[about 10 screens]. Available at URL: https://www.has-sante.fr/jcmsZc 484720/en/prise-en-charge-de-l-infarctus- du-myocarde-a-la-phase-aigue-en-dehors-des-services-de- cardiologie#ancreDocAss.

11. Appui Sante et Medico-social. Guide des bonnes pratiques organisationnelles des Centres 15 [On line]. **Agence Nationale d'Appui a la Performance des etablissements de sante et medico-sociaux, [20/10/2008];[about1 screen].** Available at URL: https://www.anap.fr/ressources/publications/detail/actualites/ameliorer- lorganisation-des-centres-15/.

12. Ministry of Health, Youth and Sport. Rapport de la mission DGOS relative a la modernisation des services d'aide medicale urgent [On line]. Ministere de la sante, de la jeunesse et des sports, [cited 13/11/2008]; [about 5 screens]. Available at URL: https://solidarites- sante.gouv.fr/IMG/pdf/circulaire 337 131108.pdf.

13. Mallouli M, Hchaichi I, Ammar A, Sehli J, Zedini C, Mtiraoui A, et al. Audit des dossiers patients d'un service mobile d'urgence et de reanimation : de l'utilité d'un référentiel tunisien. Sante Publique. 2017;(29)1:71-9.

14. Romain T. Concordance entre les diagnostics poseses a la salle d'accueil des urgences vitales et les diagnostics hospitaliers d'aval [These]. Medicine: Nancy; 2012. 121p.

15. Matuszak C, Lamy A, Thiault F, Kervella A, Kergosien, Jacquemin B et al. Impact de l'organisation sur la definition d'une profession au sein du SAMU : Le cas des assistants de regulation medicale. Revue Fran^aise des sciences de l'information et de la communication [Online]. 2016 septembre [04/07/2019];9(1):[7pages].   Disponible   al'URL: http://joumals.openedition.org/rfsic/2235.

16. Penverne Y, Jenvrin J, Debierre V, Martinage A, Arnaudet I, Bunker I, et al. Regulation medicale des situations a risque. Ann Fr Med Urgence. 2011;89(1):1015-33.

17. Poiner CN, Levine M, Shapiro N, Hantahan JP. Concordance of field and emergency department assessment in the pre-hospital management of patients with dyspnea. Prehosp Emerg Care. 2003;7(3):440-4.

18. Berthier F. Semiologie telephonique des detresses vitales reelles. Ann Fr Med Urgence. 1998;2(1):4-6.

19. Ramadanov N, Klein R, Ramadanova N, Wilhelm B. Influence of time of mission on correct diagnosis by the pre-hospital emergency physician: a retrospective study. Emerg Med Int. 2019;1(1):1-6.

20. Seyed AM, Nasiripour AA, Tabibi SJ, Masoudi I. Evaluation of emergency department performance improvement-a systematic review on influence factors. Emerg Med Int. 2016;55(1):85-100.

21. Rodriguez CG, Villar DC, Campo I. Diagnostic consistency between primary care and specialized care following emergency consultation. Atenprimaria. 2000;7(25):292-6.

22. Brunel O, Dehours E, Charpentier S, Bounes V. Comparison of the performance of an algorithm versus medical intuition in the diagnosis of non-ST+ ACS in the pre-hospital setting. Ann Fr Med Urgence. 2018;(2):87.

23. Senicourt. Concordance des diagnostics pre-hospitaliers et hospitaliers chez les patients adresses aux services d'accueil des urgences adultes de Saint Nazaire par SOS medecins : une évaluation des pratiques professionnelles [These]. Medicine: Nantes; 2016. 139p.

24. Societe Franchise de medecine d'urgence. SAMU Centre 15: new professions and new practices. Referentiel. SFMU [On line]. [cité en Mars2015];[environ 86 ecrans]. Disponible a I'URL: https: //www.samu-urgencesdefrance.fr/medias/files/155/802/sfmusudf_referentiel_samu_201 5.pdf.

25. Giroud M. La regulation medicale en medecine d'urgence. Reanimation. 2012;18:737-41.

26. Karma S, Zouari A,   Frikha M,   Dridi S,Ghanem C,   et al.   Arret cardiorespiratoire   dusujet ageen   prehospital   .   TunisMed   . 2011;89(6):529-33.

27. Jonathan RS, Fernandez R, Shimberg B, Garifo M, Correll M. The Association between emergency medical services field performance assessed by high fidelity simulation and the cognitive knowledge of practicing paramedics. Soc Acad Emerg Med [Online]. 2011 November [17/11/2011];18(11):[8]. Available at URL: https://onlinelibrary.wiley.com/doi/full/10.1111/i.1553-2712.2011.01208.x.

28. Saidi H, Hrizi L, Touihri N, Fayala R, Ben Yahya C, Gharsalli MN, et al. Jeunesse et vieillesse a travers le Recensement General de la Population et de I'Habitat 2014 [online]. Inst Nat de Sante, 2014 [cited October 2017]; [approximately 101 screens]. Disponible a I'URL: http://www.ins.tn/sites/default/files/publication/pdf/Livret-Jeunesse- oldage.pdf.

29. Rasmussen MB, Frost L, Stengaard C, Brorholt JU, Dodt K, Sondergaard HM, et al. Diagnostic performance and system delay using telemedicine for prehospital diagnosis in triaging and treatment of STEMI. Heart. 2014;100(9):711-5.

APPENDIX 1: Case Report Form (CRF)

Centre Militaire d'Aide Medicale Urgente CMAMU HMPIT	2018	Emergency Department SAU HMPIT

Study: concordance between diagnoses made by regulating physicians and
interventional physicians
versus emergency physicians
CASE REPORT FORM N°/
TO BE COMPLETED BY THE REGULATORY PHYSICIAN

DATE Patient no./Month File no.

1/ Patient details

Date of birth / Age		Gender M/F		Status MA 1 FM 2	
Address, Location of patient :					
Greater Tunis (please specify)	Bizerte	Nabeul	Zaghouan	Beja	Other (please specify)
Call time	...HH...MM	Decision -T ransfer 1 -Leave in place 2		SMUR A 1 SMUR B2	

Diagnostic suspicion after regulation (as precise as possible)
What is the relevance of your diagnosis?

Very low	Low	Average	Strong	Very strong	Certain

Emergency level :

Absolute emergency		Relative urgency	
R1	R2	R3	R4

Section 2: <u>to the SMUR emergency doctor</u>
TO BE COMPLETED BY THE SMUR DOCTOR

DATE Patient no./Month File no.

1/ Data relating to the transfer

SMUR activation time: HH MM

SMUR team

MG	
Resident	
Nurse	

Other	

Additional examinations carried out

ECG	
Dextro	
Hemocue	
HbCO	

Suspected SMUR diagnosis (as accurate as possible)

Transfer destination :

- HMPIT emergencies: (1yes /2no)
- Other HMPIT service :   (please specify)
- Other Establishment :   Department :   (please specify)

Diagnostics Group	
CCMS class	

Section 3: To be completed by the emergency department doctor
TO BE COMPLETED BY THE INVESTIGATOR IN THE HMPIT EMERGENCY DEPARTMENT

DATE Patient no./Month File no.

Triage emergency level (Canadian scale) :

T1	T2	T3	T4	T5

Care sector :

SAUV	SSR	Consultation BOX	RAD of Sorting

Exit diagnosis :

Length of stay in emergency department: (in hours/ days)

Additional examinations

Biology		Imaging	

Final patient outcome :

Resuscitation		UHCD	
Medicine (please specify)		RAD	
Surgery (please specify)		DCD	

N° Mission :
Date : --- / --- / -----   Heure : --- h ---
Permanencier : -
Médecin Régulateur : -

ANNEXE 2 : CMAMU
Fiche de Régulation Médicale

République Tunisienne
Ministère de la Défense Nationale
Direction Générale de la Santé Militaire

Ligne :
199 ☐
RIID ☐ - - - - - - - - - - - - - - - - -
Autre ☐ - - - - - - - - - - - - - - - -

Appelant :
Nom : - - - - - - -   Prénom : - - - - - - - - - -
Statut : - - - - - - - -   Tél : - - - - - - - - - - - -
Adresse : -
- -
Patient ☐   SAMU/SMUR ☐
Tierce Personne ☐   Protection Civile ☐
Médecin de Corps ☐   Police ☐
Hôpital Militaire ☐   Garde Nationale ☐
Hôpital Civil ☐   Clinique Privée ☐
MLP ☐   Autres - - - - - - - - - - ☐

Identité du Patient :
Nom : - - - - - - - - - - -   Prénom : - - - - - - - - - -
Age : - - - - - - - - - - - -   Sexe : M ☐ F ☐
Statut : - - - - - - - -   Grade : - - - - - - - - - - - -
Mle/CS : - - - - - - - - -   Tél : - - - - - - - - - - - -
Adresse : -
Rue : -
Près de : -

Lieu de l'Intervention
Domicile ☐   Hôpital ☐
Voie Publique ☐   Unité Militaire ☐
Lieu Public ☐   Cabinet Médical ☐
Lieu de Travail ☐   Clinique ☐
Autres - - - - - - - - - ☐

Nbre de Victimes : - - -

Motif de l'Appel :
Demande d'aide non méd. URG ☐
Demande d'aide méd. non URG ☐
Demande d'aide méd. URG ☐
(P0 - P1 - P2)

Interrogatoire et Pré-bilan ☐
Source de l'information :
(Patient - Appelant)

Détails du compte-rendu ☐

Décision de la Régulation :
Sortie Primaire ☐
S. Secondaire : Transfert ☐
S. Secondaire : Ex Compl ☐
S. Secondaire : Acte Spécifique ☐
Conseil médical ☐
Aviser le Médecin de Corps ☐
Vers URG par un moyen simple ☐
Indisponibilité des moyens ☐
Demande incomplète ☐
Transfert de l'appel au - - - - - - - - ☐

Véhicule engagé :
Ambulance A ☐
Ambulance B ☐
VL ☐
Autres - - - - - - - - - - - - - - - - - - - ☐

Pathologie évoquée :
Cardio-vasculaire ☐
Respiratoire ☐
Neurologique ☐
Endocrinologique ☐
Digestive ☐
Toxicologique / Intoxication ☐
Infectieuse ☐
Traumatologique / Plaie par balle ☐
Gynéco-Obstétrique ☐
Urologique / Néphrologique ☐
ORL ☐
Ophtalmologique ☐
Psychiatrique ☐
Stomatologique ☐
Autres - - - - - - - - - - - - - - - - - - - ☐

Départ de la Base : - - - h - - -   Arrivée sur les Lieux : - - - h - - -

Bilan du médecin intervenant :

Décision :
Evacuation / Transfert ☐   Annulé avant arrivée SP ☐
LSP vivant ☐   Pas de victime / Victime non vue ☐
Refus d'évacuation ☐   Evacué par propre moyen ☐
DCD sans réanimation ☐   Evacué par ambulance ☐
DCD après réanimation ☐   Evacué par PC ☐
Conseil ☐   Evacué par - - - - - - - ☐

Départ des Lieux : - - - h - -

Evolution et Suivi :
Stationnaire ☐   Aggravation ☐
Amélioration ☐   Décès ☐

Arrivée à Ets Receveur : - - - h - - -

Etablissement Receveur : - - - - - - -   Service : - - - - - - - - - - - - - - -
Régulation faite : Oui ☐   Non ☐
Médecin : - - - - - - - - - - - - - - - - - - -   Tél : - - - - - - - - - - - - - - - - - - -

Départ de Ets Receveur : - - - h - - -   Retour à la Base : - - - h - - -

Utilité de l'intervention :
Utile ☐   Inutile ☐
Mission Terminée : ☐

Appendix 3: CMAMU medical file (procedure form)

Tunisian Republic Ministry of National Defence Directorate General of Military Health	**Medical file** **CMAMU**

MISSION :

Fiche N° : Date   :   /   / PhysicianRegulator :

Intervention doctor: Nurse :

Ambulance driver :

Location :

Means of intervention: AR □ VL □ Evasan □ Reason for call :

□ Primary outing □ Secondary output (Transfer) □ Secondary output (Ex Compl) □ Secondary Output (Specialised Act)	Call time : h Base start time: h Arrival time Location: h Start time Location: h Arrival time Receiving hospital : h Receiving Hospital Departure Time: h Base arrival time: h

Requesting department: Dr :

Tel:

Receiving department: Agreement with Dr :

Tel:

PATIENT IDENTIFICATION :

Last name: First name: Sex M □ F □ Date of birth

birth date: /.../

Status: Grade: Mle / CS :

Address:

MEDICAL HISTORY :

TREATMENT IN PROGRESS :

HDM :

INITIAL CLINICAL ASSESSMENT :

Neurological :

Cardiovascular :

Respiratory :

Gastrointestinal :

Osteoarticular :

Gynecological :

Renal :

Others :

PACKAGING :

VEINOUS SURROUNDINGS				AIRWAYS			MECHANICAL VENTILATION	
A	S	Peripheral :	G	A	S	Nasal O2 :	Fashion :	
A	S	Peripheral :	G	A	S	Face mask :	Fi O2 :	
A	S	Peripheral :	G	A	S	High concentration mask :	Tidal volume :	ml
A	S	Venous KT Central :	F	A	S	Laryngeal mask n° :	Frequency :	/ min
A	S	Desilet :	F	A	S	Tracheal approach n° :	PEEP :	cm H2O

A	S	Scope	A	S	Splint	A	S	Urinary catheter :
A	S	VAC	A	S	Cervical collar	A	S	Gastric tube :
A	S	CPAP	A	S	Hard plan	A	S	Chest drain :
A	S	NIV	A	S	Shell	A	S	Other :

A: Conditioned before **S:** Conditioned by the SMUR

ECG :
MONITORING :

Time												
GCS												
TA												
FC												
FR												
SpO2												
T°												
GAD												

TREATMENT :

P	1								
E	2								
R	3								
F.	4								
Blood									
D	1								
R	2								
O	3								
G	4								
	5								
	6								
U E S	7								

RCP : ☐
DECISION :

LSP ☐ (Alive - DCD without rea - DCD after rea - Refusal to evacuate* - Medical advice)

Transport ☐

EVOLUTION :

Stationary ☐   Improvement ☐   Worsening ☐

Deaths ☐

RECEIVING INSTITUTION : ReceivingDepartment   :

Confides in Dr

DIAGNOSIS :

* This signature certifies that the patient has refused transport. Full name: N°CIN :

Signature :

CODING OF CMAMU TRANSPORT OPERATIONS

Transport No :

DIAGNOSIS :
A: Accidents and various pathologies :

I: Poisoning / Drug addiction :

☐   **I 00** Other poisoning

☐ **A 00** Other pathologies
☐ **A 01** Electrification
☐ **A 02** Hanging / Strangulation
☐ **A 03** Drowning
☐ **A 04** Hypothermia
☐ **A 05** Heat stroke / Malignant hyperthermia
☐ **A 06** Crush syndrome / Rhabdomyolysis
☐ **A 07** Burns
☐ **A 08** Allergy, Anaphylactic shock
☐ **A 09** Hypovolemic shock
☐ **A 10** Inexplicable shock
☐ **A 11** Gunshot wound / Mine explosion

C: Cardiovascular pathology :
☐ **C 00** Other cardiac pathologies
☐ **C 01** Cardiac arrest
☐ **C 02** Non-ST + coronary syndrome
☐ **C 03** ST+ coronary syndrome
☐ **C 04** Pulmonary embolism
☐ **C 05** Other chest pain
☐ **C 06** Rhythm disorders
☐ **C 07** Conduction disorders / Pace-maker
☐ **C 08** Cardiogenic shock
☐ **C 09** Hypertensive emergency
☐ **C 10** acute cardiogenic pulmonary syndrome
☐ **C 11** Vascular pathology

D: Digestive / Uro-Nephrological Pathology :
☐ **D 00** Other digestive and uro-nephro
☐ **D 01** Digestive bleeding
☐ **D 02** Acute renal failure

E: Endocrine / Metabolic pathology :
☐ **E 00** Other endocrine and metabolic disorders
☐ **E 01** Hypoglycemia
☐ **E 02** Dehydration
☐ **E 03** Acute suprarenal insufficiencyë

F: Infectious pathology :
☐ **F 00** Other infectious diseases
☐ **F 01** Septic shock
☐ **F 02** AIDS

G: Gyneco-obstetric pathology :
☐ **G 00** Other gynaeco-obstetric pathologies
☐ **G 01** GEU
☐ **G 02** Threat of childbirth
☐ **G 03** Childbirth
☐ **G 04** Eclampsia / Pre-eclampsia
☐ **G 05** Metrorragies
☐ **G 06** Abortion / Threat of abortion
☐ **G 07** Neonatal distress

☐ **I 01** Drug intoxication/Alcohol
☐ **I 02** Acute isolated drinking
☐ **I 03** Intoxication by gas, smoke (CO...)
☐ **I 04** Caustic poisoning, petroleum derivatives
☐ **I 05** Poisoning by agricultural products

N: Neurological pathology :
☐ **N 00** Other neurological conditions
☐ **N 01** H. meningee / Stroke / TIA / ICH
☐ **N 02** Convulsion / EMC
☐ **N 03** Other comas
☐ **N 04** Discomfort / Brief PC

O : Ophthalmology / ENT / Stomato :
☐ **O 00** Ophthalmological pathology
☐ **O 01** ENT pathology
☐ **O 02** Stomatological pathology

P: Pulmonary and Respiratory Pathology :
☐ **P 00** Other pulmonary and respiratory
pathologies
☐ **P 01** Asthma
☐ **P 02** Dyspnea / Acute respiratory distressë
☐ **P 03** Non-traumatic pneumothorax
☐ **P 04** lesional edema
☐ **P 05** Hemoptysis

Q : Psychiatric pathology :
☐ **Q 00** Other psychiatric conditions
☐ **Q 01** Agitation / Confusional state
☐ **Q 02** Hysteria / Simulation
☐ **Q 03** Anxiety / Anxiety attack

T : Traumatology / Orthopaedics :
☐ **T 00** Other traumatic conditions
☐ **T 01** TC insulated
☐ **T 02** Minor injury
☐ **T 03** Polycontus / Severe and/or multiple
wounds
☐ **T 04** Polyfracture
☐ **T 05** Polytrauma
☐ **T 06** Isolated limb fracture
☐ **T 07** Spinal trauma
☐ **T 08** Abdominal trauma
☐ **T 09** Pelvic trauma
☐ **T 10** Thoracic trauma
☐ **T 11** Maxillofacial trauma
☐ **T 12** Non-traumatic orthopaedic pathology
☐ **T 13** Traumatic vascular pathology

LOCATION OF INTERVENTION :	**CIRCUMSTANCES:**	**MAIN PATHOLOGY EVOQUEE:**
☐ Home	☐ Domestic accident	☐ Accidents and various pathologies
☐ Military site	☐ AVP pieton	☐ Cardiovascular pathology
☐ Public roads	☐ AVP two wheels	☐ Digestive Pathology / Uro-Nephro
☐ Public place	☐ AVP light vehicle	☐ Endocrine / Metabolic pathology
☐ Place of work	☐ AVP heavy goods vehicle	☐ Infectious diseases
☐ Place of detention	☐ AVP public transport	☐ Gyneco-Obstetric Pathology
☐ Hospital	☐ Railway accident	☐ Poisoning / Drug addiction
☐ SMU	☐ Fall from a great height	☐ Neurological pathology
	☐ Collapse of premises	

☐ Medical practice ☐ Clinic ☐ Other	☐ Fire, Explosion ☐ Accident at work ☐ Sports accident ☐ Physical aggression ☐ Stab wound ☐ Firearm wound ☐ Medical pathology ☐ Other	☐ Ophthalmology / ENT / Stomatology ☐ Pulmonary and respiratory pathology ☐ Psychiatric pathology ☐ Traumatology / Orthopaedics

SCORE DE GLASGOW (GCS) :

Ouverture des yeux (Y)	Spontanée
	Sur ordre
	A la stimulation douloureuse
	Absente
Réponse verbale (V)	Cohérente
	Confuse
	Inappropriée
	Incompréhensib
	Absente
Réponse motrice (M)	Sur ordre
	Orientée
	Evitement inadapt
	Flexion
	Extension
	Absente

GCS = ... / 15

SCORE DE MALINAS :

Score / Critères	0	1	2
Parité	1	2	> 3
Durée travail	< 3 h	3-5 h	> 5 h
Durée contractions	< 1 min	1 min	> 1 min
Intervalle	> 5 min	3-5 min	< 3 min
Perte des eaux	Non	< 1 h	> 1 h

Total = ...

-*Si Score < 5 :* Transport possible vers une maternité
-*Si Score > 6 :* Menace d'accouchement imminent

REGLE DES 9 DE WALLACE :

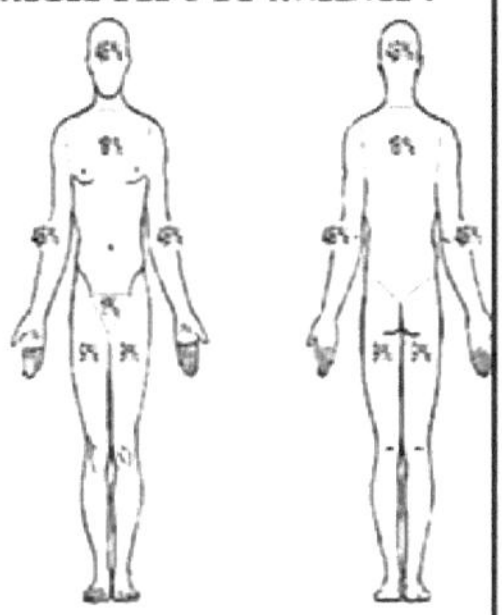

SCB : ....%
3ᵉᵐᵉ degré : ....%

Appendix 4: Classification of prioritisation by the regulatory physician

R1	Obvious or latent life-threatening emergency requiring the intervention of an emergency medical service.
R2	Emergency requiring the dispatch of a local doctor, ambulance or VSAV within the contractually agreed timeframe.
R3	Use of the permanent care service (PDS), as the delay is not a risk factor in itself.
R4	Conseil Medical.

CCMS	Definition
Class 1	Stable patient requiring no diagnostic or therapeutic procedures or on-site monitoring
Class 2	Stable patient requiring at least one diagnostic or therapeutic procedure, or on-site monitoring
Class 3	Clinical condition that can worsen without threatening life
Class 4	Immediate vital or functional prognosis without the need for life-saving treatment
Class 5	Life-threatening condition requiring vital resuscitation.
Class 6	Victim dead before the arrival of the SMUR (no resuscitation procedure undertaken)

APPENDIX 6: The Clinical Classification of Emergency Department Diseases (CCED) :

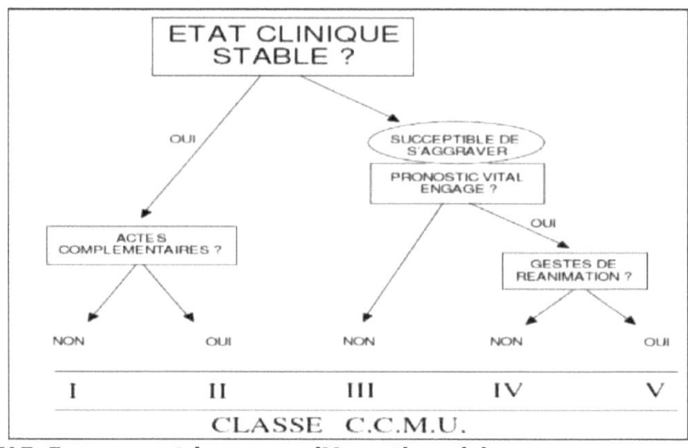

APPENDIX 7: Emergency triage score (Monastir scale)

Sorting score

SURNAME/FIRST NAME :

Variables	4	3	2	1	0	1	2	3	4
Age (ans)	-	-	-	-	< 45	45/65	66/75	76/85	> 86
Pouls	> 180	140/179	110/139	-	70/109	-	55/69	40/54	< 40
T.A.S.	> 200	-	160/199	-	80/159	-	55/79	-	< 55
Température	> 41	39/40	-	38.5/38.9	36/38.4	34/35.9	32/33.9	30/31.9	< 30
F. respiratoire	> 36	29/35	24/28	21/23	14/20	12/13	10/11	6/9	< 9
Sa O$_2$ (AA)	-	-	-	-	> 93	90/93	88/89	-	< 89
Coma Glasgow Score (CGS)	*Déficit moteur*	-	-	-	15	-	-	-	< 14
Echelle de douleur E.V.A. %	-	-	-	-	< 10	10/29	30/49	50/69	> 70

Situations particulières			
Douleur thoracique	4 Pts	Etat d'agitation	4 Pts
Perte de connaissance	4 Pts	Poly traumatisme	4 Pts
intoxication	4 Pts	Fracture ouverte	4 Pts
Brûlure ou électrocution	4 Pts	saignement	4 Pts

Patients référés	2 Pts
Antécédents	
Insuff. respiratoire/chronique/asthme	2 Pts
Insuffisance rénale chronique	2 Pts
Diabète	2 Pts
Antécédents cardiaques	2 Pts
Cirrhose	2 Pts

Appendix 8: Interpretation of the Kappa concordance index

Agreement	Kappa Index
Excellent	> 0,80
Good	0,60 < κ < 0,80
Medium	0,40 < κ < 0,60
Mediocre	0,20 < κ < 0,40
Bad	0 < κ < 0,20
Execrable	< 0

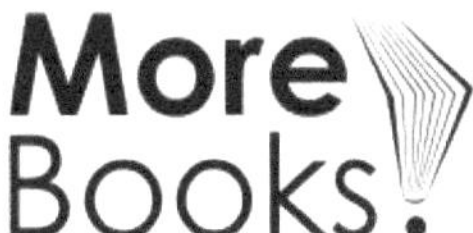

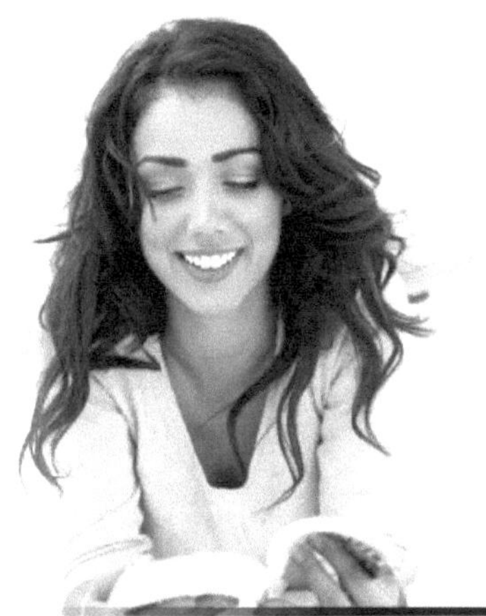

I want morebooks!

Buy your books fast and straightforward online - at one of world's fastest growing online book stores! Environmentally sound due to Print-on-Demand technologies.

Buy your books online at
www.morebooks.shop

Kaufen Sie Ihre Bücher schnell und unkompliziert online – auf einer der am schnellsten wachsenden Buchhandelsplattformen weltweit! Dank Print-On-Demand umwelt- und ressourcenschonend produziert.

Bücher schneller online kaufen
www.morebooks.shop

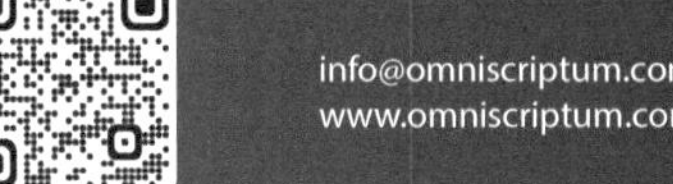

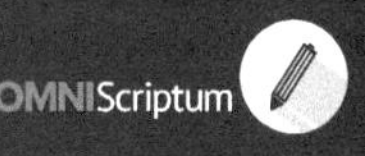

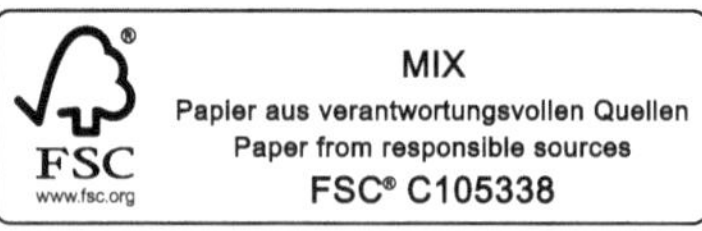

Printed by Books on Demand GmbH, Norderstedt / Germany